ALZHEIMER'S

Answers to
Hard Questions
for Families

By the same authors
The Patient in the Family

Alzheimer's

ANSWERS TO
HARD QUESTIONS
FOR FAMILIES

James Lindemann Nelson
AND
Hilde Lindemann Nelson

DOUBLEDAY
New York   London   Toronto   Sydney   Auckland

Eϵ

PUBLISHED BY DOUBLEDAY
a division of Bantam Doubleday Dell Publishing Group, Inc.
1540 Broadway, New York, New York 10036

DOUBLEDAY and the portrayal of an anchor
with a dolphin
are trademarks of Doubleday, a division of
Bantam Doubleday Dell Publishing Group, Inc.

Library of Congress Cataloging-in-Publication Data

Nelson, James Lindemann.
Alzheimer's: Answers to hard questions for families
James Lindemann Nelson and Hilde Lindemann Nelson.
p.   cm.
Includes bibliographical references.
1. Alzheimer's disease—Popular works. 2. Alzheimer's disease—
Patients—Family relationships. 3. Caregivers.
I. Nelson, Hilde Lindemann. II. Title.
RC523.2.N45   1996
382.1'96831—dc20   96-12567
CIP

ISBN 0-385-48533-6
Copyright © 1996 by the Hastings Center
All Rights Reserved
Printed in the United States of America
November 1996
First Edition

1   3   5   7   9   10   8   6   4   2

Acknowledgments

WE WROTE THIS BOOK between 1993 and 1995, when we were both employed by the Hastings Center. For going on thirty years now, the center has been a leader in the important task of trying to understand better and meet responsibly the challenges society faces from changes in medical technology and health care practice. We are grateful to our former colleagues for many kinds of assistance, and pleased that our book can claim a place in the Hastings Center tradition.

While at Hastings, our research and writing were generously supported by a grant to the center from the Greenwall Foundation. Greenwall is one of the very few philanthropic organizations to make inquiry into the ethical implications of health care a major funding priority; we appreciate its wisdom in this general respect, as well as its particular interest in our project.

We have also had the help of two kinds of consultants. One was a group of professionals in the fields of aging, elder law, social work, philosophy, and nursing home administration. We'd like to thank Marjorie Cantor, an anthropologist from the Third Age Center of Fordham University; Bartholomew Collopy, a Fordham professor of humanities, also associated with the Third Age Center; Richard T. Hull, professor of philosophy at the State University of New York at Buffalo; Harry R. Moody, the deputy director of the Brookdale Center on Aging at Hunter College; Barbara Silverstone, a social worker and president of The Light House in New York City; Peter Strauss, a lawyer specializing in elder law; Connie Zuckerman, also a lawyer and coordinator of legal studies at the SUNY Health Science Center; and most especially thanks to Tony Yang-Lewis, director of the Alzheimer's Unit at Cobble Hill Nursing Home, Brooklyn, who found most of our family caregivers for us and was invaluable in coordinating our many meetings with them. Special thanks also to Carolyn Ells, a graduate student in philosophy at the University of Tennessee, whose help was invaluable in the final stages of preparing the manuscript.

The other, even more important group of consultants was, of course, the family caregivers who advised us, told us their stories, and read every chapter, sometimes several times, pointing out where we had missed an important point or where the writing wasn't readable enough. Their stories are not the ones told here, but we could not have told these stories well without their help. To Robin Benoff, Bessie Blow, Helen Broder, Doris Brunsen, Roberta Burke, Judith Carlin, Eleanor Glass, Helen Glassman, Judy Knipe, Robert Kushner, Sylvia Mosola, Rita and Darren Pearl, Evelyn and Frank Roselle, Willie Senders, Shirley Spain, Lenore and Neil Stoller, Susan Sugarman, Catherine Unsino, Aurora and John Walton, Sandy Weisman, Paula Westho, and Howard Wolk, our deepest thanks for all your help and apologies for anything we still didn't get right. We dedicate this book to you.

HILDE LINDEMANN NELSON
JAMES LINDEMANN NELSON
Knoxville, 1996

Contents

ALZHEIMER'S

Answers to
Hard Questions
for Families

Introduction

Moral Troubles

AN EXHAUSTED, middle-aged woman stands in the bedroom doorway as the gray light of early morning outlines her father, asleep under the quilt. Barbara Kessler Johnson is just about drained. As she pulls her robe more tightly about her, she feels that with this gesture she is also holding herself together. Her dad, diagnosed several years ago as having Alzheimer's disease, is starting to stir, and she is dreading the moment when he will awake. It's not the "how-to" problems that are getting her down—how to get him to the bathroom, how to improve his appetite—it's the moral problems.

Mr. Kessler begins every morning by sitting up in bed and asking for his wife, who has been dead these twelve years. Barbara has learned the hard way that if she tells him the truth, however gently, however matter-of-factly, her father's grief will be as deep as if the loss were fresh. To him it *is* fresh, every time. Yet, if she tells a lie—if she says that her mother is out shopping, or visiting, or at work—she may have to fend off his questions all day long, piling further lies on top of the first one. Her father is not so demented that he always accepts what he's told without question; if she lies, he's likely to be suspicious and sometimes flat-out nasty, blaming his daughter for keeping his wife from him.

Barbara is profoundly tired of wrestling with this problem, and with all the other problems he causes as well. The refrain that's been running through her head for months starts up again: Dad really should be in a nursing home. But shortly after he was finally diagnosed, he asked her repeatedly to promise that she would never "turn him out of his own house." She gave him her word, and meant it. Of course, when she made that promise, Barbara didn't know what she knows now. She didn't know how hard it would be to take care of him. She didn't know that she'd be facing life without her own husband, who left her two years before to marry a woman both younger and unburdened by a demented father. And while she didn't have great hopes of her brothers, she didn't know they would leave virtually all of Dad's care to her.

As Barbara and tens of thousands of other family caregivers have discovered, a diagnosis of Alzheimer's or another dementing disease is devastating news, not only for the person suffering from it but for everyone who is "in close": spouse, children, nieces, nephews, and sometimes parents. People with these illnesses and their families feel despair and helplessness in the face of a future that seems full of terrible and altogether unavoidable problems.

Some of these problems are, of course, medical ones. Many dementias—Alzheimer's in particular—are difficult to *diagnose*. Family physicians too often pass off the symptoms of dementing diseases as "the natural effects of aging," while some victims are skillful at covering for themselves by playing down the impact of the early stages of their illnesses and, in general, helping themselves and their families to deny what they are all going through. Uninformed professionals and families in denial can conspire to keep the fundamental question, "What are we dealing with here?" waiting a long time for an answer—often, too long for the family and the patient to work out together the best ways of living with a dementing disease.

When questions about diagnosis are finally resolved, patients and families face new but equally urgent questions. What's going to happen from here on? When will it happen? How long will Mom be able to drive and to manage her own checkbook? How long can Dad continue to live independently, or to make decisions about his own health care? How long will my husband even recognize the people he has loved all his life? Is there any chance of slowing or maybe stopping the terrible destructiveness of the disease? What can medicine really do to help? Can those of us who love this person do anything? What resources are there in my community?

But when Barbara Johnson stands before her sleeping father she needs a different kind of help. She needs *moral* help. She's struggling to understand what exactly she's doing when she tells him the truth, how far she has to go to keep her promises, what adult children owe their frail and aging parents, what marriage is supposed to mean in sickness and in health, and what counts as a loving response from the rest of the family to those who do the hands-on care. All of these problems are moral ones, because they have to do with what's *right* to do, with how one *ought* to behave. And they all require active (even if temporary) solutions.

But Barbara's struggling with something else, too—something that's even harder than the solvable problems that are on her mind. She's struggling with how to live in the face of the problems she *can't* solve. And this is really the heart of the moral task that confronts her: to keep herself whole as she meets the challenge of her father's illness, without crumpling under the weight of it, without becoming hard and embittered, without protecting herself by turning away from her father's need. She has to figure out how to be faithful to her ongoing moral commitments and how to form the new ones that may be required. She has to know the difference between what can be helped and what can't, and she has to be able to revise her judgments as the disease progresses. She has to try to stand fast. For all of us, that is perhaps the most deeply moral activity. For those who have undertaken the care of a person with a dementing disease, it is also perhaps the most difficult.

This book is for Barbara and others who are struggling to be, feel, and do what is loving and responsible as they care for family members suffering from dementing diseases. It consists of stories—one to a chapter—we have created to describe what a particular family might be going through at a particular point in the progression of a dementing disease. None of the characters is intended to resemble anyone we know or have heard of, but their experiences are based on real-life stories told to us by over two dozen family caregivers, who are themselves grappling with the issues we raise here.

Stories—whether true or fictional—are always told by selecting certain details out of the vast array life lays before us, and arranging them in a way that makes sense. The stories in this book are no exception. They are told in an attempt to make sense of a crucial job families perform for their ill and, finally, dying loved ones. To make sense of that activity, however, we had to do more than *acknowledge and describe* what the Barbaras of this world are going through. We had to offer ways of *understanding* it—ideas that might be of use to busy, distressed, and sometimes exhausted caregivers who have neither the time nor the energy to sort out all these things on their own. We spent a number of years at the Hastings Center—a research institute devoted to ethical issues in medicine—thinking about what the work of caregiving means in the context of family life. In these stories, we have combined our experience as researchers with the experiences of family members who are caring for loved ones with dementia.

A word about how we use pronouns. We've tried to avoid using "he" to mean either a man or a woman. When we make a general point, we usually use "they." Where this is clumsy, we tend to use "she" in chapters where the patient is a woman, and "he" where the patient is a man.

Getting Moral Help

Family members involved in the care of a person suffering from progressive dementia may have friends, relatives, clergy, or a support group with whom they can talk over their problems—both those that must be solved and those that can't be solved—but they will find that little has been written about the most morally troubling issues of family caregiving. This book will address those problems. Here, we help people like Barbara to anticipate and carefully think through a number of the ethical concerns that surround dementing diseases, so that the anguish they *must* feel is not made worse by anguish that is *avoidable*.

In this book, we try to identify in detail the moral tasks that face family caregivers, and we offer suggestions for better ways of coping with them. But, you may ask, aren't moral tasks just the ones about which people always say, "There are no right or wrong ways to do them"? Don't they involve the most personal and individual decisions possible? Indeed they do, but that doesn't mean there are no right or wrong ways to do them, and it doesn't mean that nothing is gained by learning how others have done them.

Our moral commitments reflect something very basic about us, about who we take ourselves to be, and about our deepest hopes for ourselves, those we live with, and our world. In this respect, they are extremely individual and personal. At the same time, people's commitments are influenced by how they understand certain facts: what their options are, what ideas undergird them, and where their priorities lie. People are also influenced by other people, both those in their families and those outside them. These others will also have moral commitments that reflect *their* understanding of the options, *their* grasp of the ideas, and *their* sense of the priorities. Disagreements are possible about all these matters, but so is conversation, persuasion, give-and-take, and compromise that needn't take away anyone's integrity.

It's tempting to think that people caring for someone with a dementing disease have enough problems without having to worry about the moral niceties. Yet, just as with dementia itself, closing one's eyes to these problems won't make them disappear. We believe that they will trouble most if not all family caregivers. Our aim, then, is to provide practical, solid help to those who are thinking through and living with the ethical challenges of caring for relatives with Alzheimer's or similar diseases.

PROBLEMS TO BE SOLVED

The larger task of living through this difficult period involves solving the smaller moral problems not once but repeatedly. What was at first an adequate response can become less so as the dementia progresses, and new strategies must be found.

Family caregivers routinely have to worry about telling the truth, keeping promises, coming to grips with the meaning of serious illness, preserving the patient's dignity, and maintaining familial relationships, although they may not use the words *moral* or *ethical* to describe their problems (we'll use those words interchangeably). Some of these problems arise as dementia challenges a family's ability to care not only for the patient's body, but for something deeper, something more like the patient's "true" self. Other problems have to do with tradeoffs among competing values: the patient's safety versus the patient's independence, for example, or the familiarity of home versus the reliability of institutional care. And a final set of problems has to do with conflicts within the family—differences of opinion about what kind of care is appropriate, or the competing claims of children or spouse on the caregiver's energy and attention. The moral problems Barbara must face and must solve—sometimes repeatedly—include these:

- **How can I honor my father's dignity when he acts in ways that embarrass him or me?**

"Dignity" is a more complicated idea than we sometimes realize. When we speak of dignity, we often have two different senses of the word in mind, one having to do with *what we are* and the other with *what we can do*. The first sense reflects our feeling that we all have a certain worth—a dignity that ought to be respected by others—simply because we are people. We aren't just objects for other people to use. Dignity, however, also seems to concern our ability to do things, particularly to control our own lives in ways that are appropriate to our circumstances. Dignity in this second sense recalls the word's original Latin meaning, "fitting" or "suitable": we are meant to behave in ways that are suited to our age, gender, occupation, or social standing.

As Barbara knows all too well, a dementing disease can often involve both lapses and outbursts that seem to lessen the patient's dignity and cause embarrassment to him and those who love him. Early in his illness, her dad was deeply ashamed of forgetting people's names, and of the occasional lapses in his conversation. A very sociable person all his life, he dropped his friends like hot coals rather than suffer the indignity of having them drop him. Barbara felt that the loss of his friends was one of the worst things the disease did to him, but she didn't know what to do about his fear of losing his dignity in the eyes of his friends. Nor was she sure how she should deal with the things he did that were inappropriate to his age and social standing (and in that sense undignified) without taking away his dignity as a person.

• How can I help Dad keep a sense of himself as someone who is more than simply the victim of a dementing illness?

Having a dementing disease is a central fact in a person's life. But people are more than their diseases, and as the person's own ability to express who he is through his words and actions fades, preserving his identity becomes more and more the job of those who love and care for him. Think of what you do to a person with Alzheimer's disease when you introduce him to someone by saying, "This is Henry. Henry was a lawyer." One man who was introduced this way gently interrupted: "I *am* a lawyer." This man was fighting to maintain his sense of self—an extremely precious thing—against the incursions of his disease. Those around him missed an opportunity to be his ally in this struggle.

• How can I help my father plan for his future—a future in which decisions must be made about financial matters, medical treatment, and other issues that affect not only the person who is ill but also those whose lives are intertwined with his?

What about a "living will," or some other form of advance planning for a time when life-sustaining treatment might not be wanted? How would Barbara's dad feel about tube-feeding if he couldn't swallow anymore? And how will he and Barbara both feel if she can't continue to take care of him? How will they feel if he has to go to a nursing home?

As with any illness, managing a dementing disease involves making many decisions. These decisions are both extremely difficult and extremely important, concerning everything from how and where a person will live, to how and when death will occur. The person most affected by the decisions—the one who is ill—is less and less able to understand what is at stake, less able to form an opinion about what should be done, and less able to express that opinion, even supposing he had formed one. Barbara's father has now passed the point of being able to do any of these things—but Barbara talked to him when he still could. It was crucially important to consult him then, not only because it was his care and his life that were under discussion, but also because good advance planning was needed to relieve burdened family members of at least part of their load of grief and guilt.

• How can I give, or help my father get, the kind of care he needs right now?

Barbara needs to make sure her dad is bathed, fed, taken to the toilet; that his personal appearance is cared for. Further, she needs to ensure his physical safety while preserving such independence as he can manage. Simply finding out how to get the help that Barbara's community makes available to demented persons and their families has been a difficult responsibility for her. But whether hands-on care is provided by helpers from the community, by family members, by professionals the family has hired, or any combination of these, there remains the problem of knowing how to adjust care to the real needs of the person who is ill. Proper care for his physical well-being might require relinquishing some degree of independence in the interests of safety. Yet proper care for his dignity, for his sense of himself as a person, may require exactly the opposite tradeoff.

• **Is it ever all right to lie to demented people? Can I lie and still deserve the trust of someone who is suffering in this way? Is lying always disrespectful?**

Almost everybody, at some point in life, will avoid uncomfortable truths, "edit" their own memories, mislead others, and even sometimes tell out-and-out falsehoods. And almost everybody feels uncomfortable about lying repeatedly. As Barbara wrestles with this problem, she has put herself in her dad's shoes and acknowledged that *she* would feel very uncomfortable if it turned out that someone was lying to *her*. Even so, she also knows from experience that the price of avoiding a lie can sometimes be just as high as the price of telling one.

While people will agree that one ought to tell the truth whenever possible, it's not so easy to say precisely why that's so. To understand better whether and when it's morally okay to break the rule against lying, it's necessary to figure out just what's at stake in telling the truth or failing to do so. Once family caregivers have figured this out for a given situation, it's easier for them to see what to do.

• **What should I do if Dad asks me to help him kill himself so he can escape the worst of the disease?**

More even than the physical suffering that may accompany old age and death, many people fear the long, slow decline of their mental abilities. Pain can be alleviated with analgesics and met with a kind of noble courage; human relationships can often be maintained even if someone is suffering greatly. But dementia is different. There is no painkiller to make it go away, and in the end it takes from us even our ability to recognize those with whom we have built our lives, even our ability to recognize ourselves. In the face of this, it's no wonder that suicide appears an acceptable—perhaps attractive—option to many people. The first person Dr. Jack Kevorkian helped with his suicide machine, Janet Adkins, turned to him because she preferred death to dementia.

What should families do in the face of a loved one's desire to die? Is there anything that can be done to provide a demented person with alternatives that are attractive enough to make suicide seem undesirable? Can we, for example, distinguish between his progressive dementia, which is not curable, and his depression, which may be? Can we persuade the person that he can't lose his dignity no matter what the disease does to him? And if all attempts to safeguard the dignity of the demented person and all efforts to improve his situation fail, can we in good conscience help this person die? Can we live with ourselves if we *don't* help? How can we reconcile what suffering members of our families need from us with what we owe our consciences and the wider communities of which we are all a part?

• **How can I balance what I owe to my own children and my spouse against the increasingly heavy burden of caring for my demented father?**

As if walking one tightrope at a time isn't hard enough, family caregivers have to walk a number of them all at once. They must skillfully weigh the conflicting needs and interests of the person who is ill, but they also have to respond to the needs, desires, interests, and claims of other family members.

Barbara's husband didn't feel she was doing a good job of this. If you asked him, he would say he left because Barbara's devotion to her father was eating up so much of her time and attention that it effectively ended their relationship. He believes she showed by the choices she made that her marriage wasn't very important to her. Barbara herself, of course, looks at it differently: she thinks George kept his promise to be faithful "for better," but lacked the integrity to hang in there "for worse." Regardless of who is right, there are times when she feels not only angry at her husband for letting her down but angry at herself for allowing so much of her life to be consumed by her father's care.

What do we owe our children or our spouses, and how stringent are those obligations? And how should we resolve disagreements among family members about sharing the burdens of care? Just as it's important to talk with the person facing dementia about his future care, so too is it important for family members to talk among themselves about how to divide the tasks of care. Many important differences and old resentments are apt to surface when families get together and talk about which people are and which aren't doing their share, so these conversations can be dangerous. What can be done to make them productive rather than damaging?

· How can I take care of myself when I'm so busy responding to everyone else's needs?

It sometimes seems as if caregiving is a zero-sum game in which those who get the care take away from those who give it, leaving the caregiver empty and drained. Part of the balancing act is to make sure caregivers include themselves in the care they give others. How can they do this without being selfish? Where's the fine line between taking one's own needs and interests too seriously and not taking them seriously enough?

In the course of caring for her dad, Barbara discovered something that other people in her situation have noticed too: providing intensive amounts of care for someone else can enlarge your capacity to care. It can change your priorities, make certain things seem trivial that used to matter a great deal, increase your sense of the ill person's importance and value. It can make you a stronger and better person. It can also, of course, leave you irritable and mean-spirited.

What personal resources can caregivers muster to meet the demands of life more gracefully? What habits of character can they cultivate that will allow them to avoid feeling constantly angry and resentful, or hopeless and overwhelmed? And how does the progression of the dementing disease prompt caregivers to alter their strategies for self-care as time goes on?

• **When the demented person is not my parent but my spouse, how does this change the kind or quality of the care I give, and how does giving this care change me?**

Ordinarily, different people in the family will need different amounts of familial care. If needs are equal and in conflict, who gets what? Should our ill spouses win out over our children? Should parents lose out to ill husbands or wives? Should you encourage your children to help you with your spouse's care, even if they have small children of their own? And even if we are able to answer these questions, how can we tell if needs are "equal" or not?

• How can family members resolve, or at least live with, disagreements over who will give care, the type of care, and how much it will cost?

Different family members see things differently. They often disagree about how much direct involvement in the care of a relative is necessary or desirable, and these disagreements can damage what once were loving relationships. What Barbara's dad really needed, for instance, and even how sick he was, became matters about which Barbara and her former husband very definitely didn't see eye to eye. And as if that weren't bad enough, Barbara's older brother, Bob, also thought she often overstated how sick Dad was. Such differences can lead to serious problems within the family. Some of these disagreements will come out of long-standing interpersonal issues—for example, the resentment Bob felt because Barbara was Dad's favorite child. Other disagreements arise when family members come to terms with dementia at different speeds and in different ways.

Regardless of their origin, however, these differences can become moral differences. People have different ideas about what adult children in general owe their parents, and even more, about what specific children owe their parents. When Barbara presses her brothers for more help, she runs into both these problems. Rick says she's foolish to spend so much of her life caring for Dad now that he really can't tell whether he's living at home or in a long-term care facility, while Bob nurses the aforementioned grudge, saying that since Dad never had any time for him when he was a kid, he's not going out of his way to help him now. For her part, Barbara feels exploited by both these attitudes, and her relationship with her siblings has gotten pretty rocky. She is becoming more and more isolated from her family as well as her friends.

The tasks involved in caring for demented people are burdensome enough without costing caregivers some of their most precious possessions— good relationships with people they have known and loved all their lives. Yet it can be terribly hard to discuss such difficult matters in ways that are productive, practical, and healing, rather than divisive.

• How can I keep my memories of Dad in happier days from being blotted out by how he looks and acts now?

Dementia takes away the ill person's past as it erases the memories that meant so much to him, that are so much a part of who he is. It also takes away his future, foreshortening life and destroying anticipation. These losses threaten not only the person with the disease but also those who love and care for him. The weight of caregiving may be so great and the changes so deep that a loving spouse or child loses sight of the person being cared for. Not only can the incessant demands of the day interfere with one's ability to see past the patient's needs to his *current,* still valuable self but that neediness can make it difficult to keep a vivid sense of who he *used to be,* and of how things were in the good times. When the past slips away, it takes with it a future in which these memories might continue to console and enrich us.

Barbara has struggled to hold on to her image of her father. She always saw him as a somewhat shy, soft-spoken man who seemed at the same time trustworthy, loving, strong, and essentially independent. Now he has become loud, sometimes vulgar, self-centered, and essentially dependent on her. Remembering her dad as he was has not been easy, and as that memory slips away, she is sometimes furious that she's been trapped into doing so much for a nasty stranger. And then, of course, she feels very guilty about her anger. How can she better come to terms with these feelings? What are the beliefs—about her dad, about her duties, about herself and the rest of the family—that go hand in hand with her feelings?

WHEN THE PROBLEMS CAN'T BE SOLVED

How tough is a human self, and how bad do things have to be for a caregiver before she begins to disintegrate? When we enter the world as infants, our personalities are fluid, open to being shaped by all kinds of social forces, including, most importantly, our interactions and relationships with the people who are nearest to us. The basic structures of our personalities become set in late childhood, perhaps around the age of eight or ten, by which time we have acquired defense mechanisms, a set of strategies for dealing with people, and a sense of our own identity. Our adult lives are spent refining, rather than radically altering, the person who emerges from childhood.

As we continue to interact with the world, our personalities generally remain stable, but while they may be relatively tough, they are far from immune to the blows of illness or misfortune. When those blows are inflicted repeatedly and the person lacks adequate social and emotional support, her identity begins to crumble around the edges. In extreme cases, as when a person is held hostage by terrorists or undergoes sustained torture, her personality can even shatter. If, as folk wisdom has it, suffering builds character, it is also true that too much suffering damages it. As Barbara pulls her robe more tightly about her in the early morning light, she is expressing a very real need to hold herself together during this difficult time in her life.

What will she have to do if she is to keep herself from crumbling, or becoming embittered, or retreating into indifference? Many things, not the least of which is cultivating courage and a sense of humor. But in this book we are going to pay close attention to three tasks in particular that have a special moral force. The first is staying true to oneself. The second is accepting gracefully what can't be changed. The third is seeing things clearly.

Staying true to yourself is a way of protecting your moral center—that core of values, beliefs, and commitments that are *your* way of being in the world. It's a kind of moral steadiness, which allows others to depend on you, not only on a day-to-day basis or in the long run, but also when—as in Barbara's case—push comes to shove and your ability to rise to the occasion is put to the test. Being true to yourself doesn't mean you won't have lapses—occasional outbursts of bad temper, carelessness, or egotism. It *does* mean that you don't lose sight of who you are. You keep your central values, beliefs, and commitments from shriveling up or seeping away.

Standing fast allows you to resist the twin temptations of avoidance and denial. For many of us, becoming demented is our worst nightmare—just barely edging out the fear that it might happen to someone we dearly love. We avoid what we fear, and fear feeds denial. However silly it may sound, all of us are capable of supposing that if we pretend something very disagreeable isn't there, it might just go away. Denial of dementia is all the more tempting because the symptoms that show up first aren't easy to distinguish from the common stereotypes of old age. For the longest time Barbara, her dad, and the rest of the family took refuge in the fact that Mr. Kessler had always been a little absentminded. "Everyone forgets," after all, and "it's only natural to grow a little vague as you get on in years." For months everyone in the family repeated these phrases as if they were magic.

While such denial can be an important psychological coping mechanism, it also lets us avoid responding to another person's very real needs. For Barbara this avoidance was only temporary, but for her husband it was more than that. If Barbara's judgment of him is correct, he let some core commitments slip away. He didn't stand fast. From one's own perspective, letting go of core commitments amounts to betraying something important about oneself. From the perspective of others, it means one can't be trusted. That's how Barbara's husband seemed to her.

If staying true to yourself is like courage in that it gives you the strength to do what must be done, accepting what you can't change is something like a sense of humor: it's an attitude that helps when nothing *can* be done. It's a quiet daily going on unhampered by fantasies of fixing everything or making up for it all somehow.

This kind of acceptance isn't the same as hands-in-your-lap resignation—it's not a passive enduring. It's just the opposite. It takes an active, continually revised understanding of what must now be. This kind of acceptance is what keeps us from a self-glorifying but useless martyrdom. It lets us see the limits not only of what can be done but of what *we* can do.

For Barbara, the struggle to accept gracefully what she couldn't change began with a whole lot of useless regret. Why hadn't she taken that trip with Dad ten years ago, when he was still in good health? Why had she been so impatient with him when she was going through her divorce? And for that matter, if she had only been kinder and more attentive to her husband when she first started caring for her father, maybe things would have worked out differently and she'd still be married. "What if?" "If only," and "It might have been" ran round and round in a continual refrain as she tried to come to terms with the damage her father's illness had inflicted on her own life. What Barbara had to learn was a different, less self-absorbed way of being.

Standing fast and graceful acceptance both depend on seeing clearly. It is clear-eyed perception that allows you to see not only when and how to respond but also the limits to response. It's the ability to grasp the seriousness of what you have to deal with, a capacity for estimating repairs, a shrewdness about your own strengths and weaknesses. It's a way of paying attention.

Her ability to see clearly is what allows Barbara to hold fast to her commitments, her values, her attitudes—central features of her moral identity. The shrewdness that keeps her from fooling herself, that puts the brakes on wishful thinking or self-indulgence, is what made it possible for her to let go of the idea that her dad was just becoming a little forgetful, which in turn permitted her to start meeting his needs rather than avoiding them. Likewise, her ability to see that she is not a superwoman helped her to stop scrambling repeatedly through vain regrets. The insight that she's just Barbara, warts and all, led her to understand that she doesn't have to be so sorry she didn't do everything just right, and she doesn't have to be perfect now.

1

Coping with the Early Stages

MARY O'KEEFE is fifty-seven, but she could easily pass for ten years younger. After spending her youth and her early middle age as a full-time homemaker, she's devoted the last decade to becoming a professional caterer—a lifelong ambition. She takes a deep satisfaction in being able to express herself through her cooking and prizes her independence even more than she thought she would, especially since catering has finally started to pay her a reasonably comfortable income.

One helping of love for what you do combined with a dollop of personal pride turned out to be a good recipe for staying vigorous and fresh. Ms. O'Keefe has been through a lot in her life—a nasty divorce and a bout with breast cancer—but lately she's been relaxed, confident, and successful, and the people closest to her have tended to smile when they think about how nicely her life has come together.

That's why it wasn't just devastating but also painfully ironic when the symptoms started showing up. Ms. O'Keefe rattled her daughter Janet when she put the mail in the refrigerator one day. And because it was so completely out of character, she worried her friends when she began to be late for appointments because she somehow lost her way.

But if her friends thought these episodes were cause for concern, Ms. O'Keefe thought they were horrifying and absolutely intolerable. She couldn't stand the embarrassment. Besides, she didn't want her "lapses" to upset her friends and acquaintances any more than they already had. So quietly that most of them failed to notice at first, she began to turn down their invitations and to spend more and more time at home. She simplified her catering menus and started finding reasons to refuse jobs. In short, she began to cut the ties that connected her to the life she loved.

She couldn't, however, avoid Janet, who had been living with her mother since her own recent divorce. But she's done her best to avoid situations in which Janet might have to "make allowances" for her. Unfortunately and inevitably, her best hasn't been quite good enough, and Janet has had to make adjustments to the changes in her mother's abilities. Things have now reached the point where these allowances and excuses are becoming second nature to Janet—so much so, in fact, that most of the time she hardly notices she's making them. For the last several months Janet's convinced herself (almost) that there isn't anything really so odd about Mom's behavior. She firmly believes this—except perhaps late at night, when she wakes, worries, and finds it hard to go back to sleep.

As Ms. O'Keefe has less and less to do with people outside her home, she grows more and more dependent on Janet to fulfill her needs for companionship. Janet too is seeing less of her friends. She's not as likely to go out in the evenings. Even long-distance phone calls with her sister Pam and her brother Nicholas and their families, which used to be a weekly routine, have fallen off. Like her mother, Janet is losing some of her own connections with life. More and more often she feels as if she can't go on, and she finds herself standing in front of the window display at work staring at nothing, her mind as blank as her morning. Alzheimer's disease is starting to claim more than one victim in this home.

Our job in this chapter is to examine some of the difficulties that confront families at the onset of Alzheimer's or other dementing diseases, looking to the experiences of the O'Keefe family for examples, encouragement, good ideas, and warnings. In many ways, of course, the O'Keefes' story will be unique to them. Other families will have to deal with different problems and will have different strengths and weaknesses. But every family in this situation faces some of the same challenges the O'Keefes are facing, and it can be useful to know not only what those are, but what people have done to meet them. In particular, as we think about life with the O'Keefes, we want to look at how families make the early stages of dementia even worse than they have to be, what an admirable response for this particular family might be, and what can be done when others aren't responding so admirably.

MAKING IT WORSE

Far from being ready to accept her illness, Ms. O'Keefe tried to cover up the early changes she was going through—and her children and friends tried to follow her lead. It was well over a year before she, her family, or even her doctor were ready to put a name to what was happening. And even when she was forced to acknowledge that she was ill, she still tried to hide what was happening to her—and so to hide herself—for as long as she could.

It would be better for Ms. O'Keefe if she could be more matter-of-fact about what she's losing, more willing to assert her remaining powers, and more relaxed about her new needs. That means it would be better if those who love and live closely with her could help to create a setting in which she finds it as easy as possible to *be* matter-of-fact, assertive, and relaxed. There is a lot they are all going to have to go through, a lot they have to learn and decide, and life will be easier if they can learn, decide, and go through as much as possible together. The trouble is, everyone is shrinking from meeting the problem straight on.

For some people, uncertainty is unbearable. Facing what Ms. O'Keefe faces, people who need to know where they stand would want to do all they could to get rid of the question marks, even if that meant certain knowledge that they had an incurable and progressive disease. But for other people, the very fact that this diagnosis is so threatening makes uncertainty look pretty good in comparison. People who can't stand too much reality might be relieved if their family doctor happened not to find anything wrong. They would push away the knowledge, if they had it, that Alzheimer's disease is notoriously difficult to diagnose. This kind of person wouldn't go out of her way to consult a neurologist or geriatric psychiatrist for a second opinion. There would be an overwhelming temptation to chalk the trouble up to fatigue, or stress, or simple old age.

When Ms. O'Keefe finally did receive her diagnosis, there was nothing even remotely matter-of-fact about her response. The news signaled to her the end of everything she had built her life around and everything she had aimed it toward. Her sensitivity about her privacy, her fastidious personal habits, her relationship to her family and friends, her career as a caterer—all were in jeopardy. And she couldn't turn to her loved ones and closest friends to help her face this danger, because she felt not only a crushing sense of loss but an equally crushing sense of shame.

KEEPING UP APPEARANCES

Janet's sister Pam and brother Nicholas, along with their own spouses and children, had a hard time understanding what was happening to Ms. O'Keefe. It took them longer than it took Janet to catch on, because their mother managed to do a superb job of keeping up appearances during the quarter of an hour or so each week when they spoke with her on the phone. And because *they* didn't want anything major to be the matter either, they weren't able to take Janet's worrying seriously for quite a long time. This, of course, made Janet feel there must be something wrong with *her* if she could be imagining such a frightening illness for her own mother.

Getting a reasonably firm diagnosis at this point could actually have helped Janet, because she wouldn't have felt so isolated from Pam and Nicholas and their families. Instead, she tried to keep telling herself she was just being an alarmist. She scolded herself for being too impatient with her mom, for exaggerating every little lapse, for being hypercritical. And then, of course, she stopped being "hypercritical" by trying not to notice, and that became easier the longer she pretended. So Janet too was keeping up appearances. It became a game that everyone in the family could play.

COOPERATING WITH DEMENTIA

Although Ms. O'Keefe is so humiliated and embarrassed by her illness that she pretends nothing is wrong, there is no reason for her to feel ashamed. And it's certainly not sensible for her to shrink away from the most important aspects of her life. Her strategies—not thinking about it and keeping up appearances—are actually denying her the very things she fears the disease will take away later. Cooperating with the disease in this way is becoming completely self-defeating.

It's just as unreasonable—and self-defeating— for Janet to go along with this pattern of denial and withdrawal. For months, she's used up a lot of energy trying to beat down the gnawing feeling that something is badly wrong, and in the process she is neither giving nor getting as much help as she could. Mother and daughter together are settling into a pattern that makes every day a burden. Worse still, they are doing their best to guarantee an unbearable future.

In pointing this out, we don't mean to be hard on Ms. O'Keefe, Janet, or the rest of the family. Only someone with no imagination could fail to sympathize with the O'Keefes' barrage of conflicting feelings or their temptation to bury their heads in the sand. Nevertheless, this is an absolutely crucial turning point in their shared life. For now, Ms. O'Keefe retains the mental ability to understand what is happening to her. If she has any desire to help her family respond to her illness in the way she thinks is most fitting, she had better do it while she still can.

There's still time for her to help Janet and the rest of the family work out a better understanding of what is likely to happen, what help she will need, and what role they can play in getting that help to her. Even more important, there's still time to help the family begin as they ought to go on—namely, to think of their mother not just as a burdensome responsibility, but as a *person* who has her own thoughts and feelings, her own ideas about the overall shape she wants her life to take. But because Ms. O'Keefe is pretending nothing's wrong, she's denying herself an important capacity her illness hasn't touched yet—the capacity to participate actively in plans for her future.

Janet and the rest of the family, for their part, could be helping their mother with the very difficult job of accepting the changes in her life, so that she might respond to her last illness with the courage and dignity she's always displayed in hard times. They could also be helping each other in this task of acceptance. They could be getting as clear as possible about just what problems are looming ahead, what Mom wants done about them, and what they, individually and as a family, feel they can do to meet her needs. These are things they all have the mental ability to do. But in order to start doing anything, they first have to stop cooperating with the dementia.

For a while, it didn't look as if either Mary O'Keefe or her family would be able to stop doing that. Helping one another to face the future requires the whole family to talk about what's happening, but this requirement crashes right into the wall of silence that Ms. O'Keefe and her loved ones have built around her illness. People can be very ingenious at denying to themselves what everyone else knows to be true. Denial can be a useful, even unavoidable coping device. It gives people a chance to protect their own sense of self as they gradually absorb the implications of bad news. But denial also carries real dangers, because trying not to know about a disaster often makes things much worse.

AN ADMIRABLE RESPONSE

How can people get through denial soon enough to respond constructively to a new situation?

Working through denial can be helped by professional counselors, and if a family is in a position to get this kind of help, they should consider doing it. But denial—at least the kind Ms. O'Keefe is experiencing—has ethical as well as psychological elements, and we want to explore some of these here.

SHAME

Why is Ms. O'Keefe ashamed of herself? Feeling shame involves believing that you have done something for which you can be blamed. But surely, no reasonable person could think that Ms. O'Keefe's dementia is in any sense her fault.

Unfortunately, what we actually *believe* and what we can give *good reasons for believing* aren't always the same. The shame Ms. O'Keefe feels comes out of a pretty realistic notion of how her family and friends will react when they learn about her dementia. What she really dreads, perhaps as much as anything else that may happen to her, is that they will push her outside the circle. Inside the circle is the place for "us"—we who are lucky enough to be healthy and normal, at least for the moment. Outside is the place for "them"—those who are not healthy, not normal, and therefore not really a part of things. Very important things, like the community, the family, "life."

There is nothing crazy about Ms. O'Keefe's fear. To a greater or lesser degree, many of her friends and loved ones will think, feel, and act exactly the way she's afraid they will. But the *shame* comes from the fact that Ms. O'Keefe *herself* believes she is no longer "us" but "them." This belief is damaging and it can't be justified. It can also be hard to get rid of.

Sad though it is, when a person is seen as "abnormal"—particularly if the abnormality has to do with memory or intelligence—many of us become very uncomfortable and want to avoid that person. Even sadder, the person who is uncomfortable and the person who is "abnormal" can—like Ms. O'Keefe—be the same person. This discomfort is perfectly natural. It isn't something that Ms. O'Keefe has purposely set out to feel, after all. But it is important to see that a moral judgment is playing an important role in this feeling. At some level, Ms. O'Keefe believes that ill people really are somehow made less important, less worthy, by their physical or mental limitations. They suffer a loss of status, a lessening of their dignity.

Human beings are complicated creatures, and many other beliefs may be compounding the one that says the sick are less worthy. For example, many of us have the totally mistaken but deep-rooted belief that if you avoid a person with dementia, you can lower the odds that you too will end up that way. Avoiding the person who is ill makes her feel even more unworthy, even more unlovable and isolated. Everyone in the family—

including the person with the dementia—needs to be aware that such shaming and avoidance can happen. They need to hang on to the knowledge that the disease does not make the sick person less worthy of love and respect, nor does it justify turning the person into a moral outcast.

Janet didn't have access to a professional counselor at this point; she couldn't afford it for herself, and getting her depressed mother into a therapist's office was more than Janet could handle. What she did have was the ability to examine her own feelings. She first learned how to do this when she was taking acting lessons, and she's had a lot of practice since then. Even so, it was tough for Janet to admit to herself that one of the reasons she was helping her mother avoid the truth was that she was ashamed to see this woman she loved and respected turn into "a senile old lady."

Once she admitted that, she no longer needed to hold on to the beliefs that were making her ashamed of her mother. You can't always keep nasty ideas from flying into your head, but, as Martin Luther once said, you don't have to let them build nests in your hair. So Janet started to act in ways that expressed the attitude she wanted to have. She behaved as though her mother's condition was nothing to be ashamed of, and little by little she found that the unwanted beliefs had less influence over her feelings. Janet's taking the lead in this way helped both Ms. O'Keefe and the rest of the family recognize and begin to overcome their own sense of shame.

Shame wasn't the only emotion the family had to overcome if they were to respond admirably to Ms. O'Keefe's illness. Fear is another powerful emotion, and it too can feed denial. While shame about dementia is based on beliefs that most of us would be hard-pressed to defend, fear makes much more sense. Ms. O'Keefe believed that she had a lot to be afraid of, and she was right. However, denial and avoidance, if they are at all prolonged, not only *add* to the list of problems people have to fear, but reduce the resources they have for dealing with those problems. Our very fear of dementia is, indeed, one of the things about it we most have to fear, because it can get in the way of creative and imaginative responses.

Fear can also get in the way of some very practical and straightforward responses. Medical treatment can, for example, sometimes clear up temporary dementias and minimize the symptoms of other conditions that often coexist with progressive dementias. Diseases like Alzheimer's are frequently accompanied by other mental and emotional problems, such as hallucination or depression, that can be successfully treated. The dementia itself may be made worse by physical conditions—for example, not having enough to eat or drink—that doctors can diagnose and do something about.

Fear is treacherous from a practical point of view because it delays people from getting help. Victims of dementia and those who care for them are in for the duration, and it is foolish to make life harder in the long run for what are often illusory advantages up front. But aside from this practical point, fear is also *morally* treacherous, because it produces lies and deceitful evasion. As a general rule, it's wrong to lie, because it's manipulative and disrespectful and puts the person being lied to at an unfair disadvantage. It takes away that person's freedom.

There are other opinions about lying, of course. Some people have even argued that the most moral thing to do is to deceive dementia patients about their diagnoses. A few years ago, Dr. George Markle, a physician from New Mexico, wrote a letter to the *New England Journal of Medicine* (11 March 1993) concerning his wife's death from Alzheimer's disease:

> When it became clear that my wife had Alzheimer's disease, I decided to tell her that she had a condition of forgetfulness and that she was no more to blame than a person with heart disease or arthritis. I shielded her from television programs and articles

that discussed her dismal future. While still rational, she went along with making a living will and giving me power of attorney because I did the same at the same time for her. There was therefore no reason to cause her to suffer the dreadful anticipation that she would otherwise have had to bear.

Dr. Markle went on to say that there was no medical reason for his wife to know her diagnosis. If she'd had cancer, she would have had to be told so that she could cooperate with her treatment, but since there is nothing that could have been done to stop her Alzheimer's disease, there was no point in telling her she had it.

Dr. Markle is fairly representative of people who think it's kinder not to tell the truth to those who are ill with a dementing disease, since medicine has nothing to offer them. But this is a mistake. As we have been trying to show, there is much that *can* be done, medically and morally, to help these people and their families. Besides, there's a real question as to whether the strategy that Dr. Markle tried with his wife can succeed. It would never have worked with Ms. O'Keefe, who had already seen the television shows and read the magazine articles, and who knew full well what she was afraid and ashamed of. It's likely, of course, that Ms. Markle had seen them too. If so, her husband's attempt to shield her would have been the very thing that prevented her from receiving the comfort she could otherwise have gotten. It would have prevented her from putting a name to what she feared and from sharing her troubles with the person she loved best.

In the O'Keefe family, the real moral question wasn't so much *whether* to seek out information about the symptoms that might indicate a progressive dementia, nor whether such information should be withheld from Ms. O'Keefe or soft-pedaled; it was rather *how* she should be helped through the shame and fear that were fueling her denial, and how information about her diagnosis and prognosis should be shared. We believe that these will be the real moral questions for many other families as well.

USING THE FAMILY'S IMAGINATION

Like many family caregivers in the midst of working out their own feelings, Janet will also be supporting and sustaining her mother: helping her to face the fact that her disease is progressive, incurable, and ultimately fatal; easing her shame and fear; covering up for her in social settings. She'll be doing a lot of this on her own, since Pam and Nicholas live far away. She will likely be learning what doctors can do, what kinds of day care facilities exist in her community, what kinds of long-term care options are available, what kind of coverage Medicare provides, and, in general, how to mediate between the person with dementia and the system.

Doing this well requires an active—and precise—imagination. For example, if you overestimate the degree of confusion the person with dementia is experiencing, you're apt to become overprotective and so threaten the patient's sense of independence and self-respect. On the other hand, if you underestimate the person's burden and sense of loss, you're apt to provide too little support and so increase the patient's isolation.

Janet felt she should also be careful about her own needs for support and connection—needs that would continue throughout her mother's illness. Being a sociable person at heart, she decided to seek out others who were facing the same problems. She hoped that a network of this kind would provide an opportunity for emotional support, for feedback, and for new solutions. It was a way, she thought, to profit from other people's imaginations. She called the Alzheimer's Association.

That's how she got to know Kathy and Dwayne Bailey. Martha Bailey, Dwayne's mom, had lived in a retirement home for several years and was fairly content there. This past year, however, it became clear that she couldn't live on her own much longer, and because Dwayne was the only one of her four children who lived nearby, he was by default the person in charge. He and Kathy cleaned out their guest bedroom, moved his mom into their home, and had been looking after her for the last six months.

"Our house was the logical place for her and we're glad she's with us," Kathy told Janet, "but Dwayne's brothers took it all so much for granted that it made Dwayne mad. He felt like they were too offhand about pushing all the responsibility for his mom onto us, just because we were close by and they weren't. And you know, when we talked to other people in our situation, we found out it's completely typical—one person in the family is the designated caregiver and everybody else drops out. But Eddie only lives an hour away, and Terry and Tom aren't that much farther. And Dwayne and I don't *want* all the responsibility."

Janet didn't either. "So what did you do?"

"I didn't. Dwayne did it. He invented something he calls the Family Huddle. He called his brothers on the phone and told them he didn't want them to take it for granted that his mom's care was up to him. He said he wants them to help him plan for her future. He wants them to make decisions with him about how to keep her active and interested in life, and about handling her money. He thinks they should figure out together when and if she'll need to be in a nursing home, and worry about her heart condition and all the rest. He was so sure they'd blow him off he nearly didn't call them, but he really didn't want us to have to handle this all by ourselves. So it seemed like it was worth a try."

"Did it work?" Janet asked.

"Mixed results," Kathy said wryly. "Eddie and Terry saw his point. They hadn't meant to duck out on helping—they just took it for granted that there wasn't anything for them to do, since she was living with us. Once Dwayne came up with some suggestions, like having Eddie get her to an elder care lawyer, having Terry spell us over Memorial Day weekend so we can go out of town, and having a Family Huddle on the phone once a month to sort out any problems that come up and make plans, they were surprisingly good about it. Dwayne has to take the initiative, but they're all on e-mail, and once he figured out how to set up a computer conference, he started scheduling one every month and they've had five in a row now."

"What about his other brother?"

"Oh well—he's being a jerk. But he was always a jerk, so at least he's consistent. He doesn't even come to see her. Says it makes him feel uncomfortable and that he's too softhearted to be able to stand it. Softhearted. Isn't that a great way to keep your caring, sensitive-guy credentials? We had to write him off, but then, we'd come close to writing them all off, and it's a good thing we didn't. Dwayne gets all the credit for being mad and doing something about it. But he didn't see why on earth one kid should have to shoulder all the worry."

Janet didn't see why either. Impressed by the Baileys' imaginative solution, she resolved to make her own attempt at a Family Huddle.

Family Fights

A family's task at this early stage can be very hard. There may be conflict: when some family members want to keep the diagnosis from the ill person but others don't; when, like Ms. O'Keefe, that person struggles to cover up losses and refuses to acknowledge her problem, but the family wants to break through this denial; when the person with dementia balks even at attempts to get a diagnosis; or when family members themselves move through their own denial at different rates.

The O'Keefes didn't do any better than most families at dealing with these problems. True to her resolve, Janet tried regular Family Huddles with her brother and sister. Unlike the Baileys, the O'Keefes aren't all on e-mail, but Janet found out from her telephone company how to set up a conference call and they've been having them regularly. Sometimes these conversations are emotionally exhausting for everybody. There's a tendency to revert to the kind of sniping, arguing, and put-downs the three of them used to engage in when they were kids. Nicholas gets sullen; Janet gets shrill. Pam, who's the oldest, gets unbearably bossy. Janet and Nicholas think Pam's husband doesn't treat her very well. Pam and Nicholas disapprove of a number of things Janet has done in her life. Janet and Pam are jealous of the favoritism their mother sometimes shows Nicholas. These and other undercurrents get mixed up in their discussions about their mother, not only putting the discussions in jeopardy but also putting a strain on the bonds of sisterly and brotherly love.

Just as Janet had to work hard to understand herself better and to wrestle with what she learned, so the family as a whole needs to undergo a process of self-exploration and self-education. They need to know more about their own thoughts and feelings concerning dementia— thoughts they accumulated over the years when they didn't think it would involve them directly. They need to develop a realistic view of what they will be facing in the future. They need to learn as much as they can about the resources available to them. They need to become as flexible and creative as they can.

But, as Janet has just started to realize, they need something else, too—each other. There are some practical considerations here. As the daughter who lives with their mother, Janet will, at least for the time being, have to take on the brunt of caring for her. That's a problem, because Janet was hoping to take only temporary sanctuary with her mother after the divorce. At some point she'll need her personal freedom if she's going to make new friends and trade in her dead-end job at the mall for an acting career. Pam and Nicholas have young children at home, but Janet does need them to help her as much as they can. Besides, at this stage it isn't so much the hands-on care as the *responsibility* that Janet needs to share. If she can know her brother and sister are participating in the emotional and logistical adjustments that have to be made, and that they'll stand by her when things get tougher, the illness won't be so hard to face.

Janet thinks that Pam and Nicholas need their mother too. If they detach themselves from this illness, if they let disagreements about her care serve to justify their backing off altogether, they will have lost out on a crucial opportunity to demonstrate that their relationship with their mother isn't just one of convenience and use.

This is worth thinking about for a minute. Because she was a good parent, Ms. O'Keefe provided little Pam, Nicholas, and Janet with all kinds of things, ranging from food and clothing to lessons in behavior to love. But the love she gave them when they were little wasn't like a hot meal on the table or clean laundry in the drawer—it was a *relationship,* and one the children needed to be in if they weren't going to grow up badly broken. Love has to be given as well as received: when your mom is loving you, she's teaching you to love her back. In this respect, learning to love is like learning to talk. You practice by imitating someone who knows how, and before you know it, you're in a conversation. Before Pam, Janet, and Nicholas knew it, they were in a loving relationship. They were speaking as well as hearing love, and the older they grew, the more mature their own loving became.

Loving and being loved leave you vulnerable. You're open with people you love, and that means they can hurt you far more than a stranger can. If Pam and Nicholas withdraw from their mother, not because of anything she did to deserve it but just because things are tough, they'll hurt her terribly. She's likely to feel her kids are showing that, all along, they've just been using her for the clean laundry and hot meals, that it was never really a loving relationship at all. And she'll be right. That's what Janet means when she says that Nicholas and Pam need their mother. They need her because they do love her; they aren't just in this for what they can get out of her. If ever there was a time to demonstrate their love, it is now.

So the children have a good reason to hang together even when they're furious with one another, because sharing these hard times can water and feed the whole family. Doing as much as possible together can strengthen the relationships among them, help ensure that tasks are divided fairly, and provide more clarity about the sources of their friction and disagreements. A shared commitment to seeing this through as a family is a pledge that no one will abandon the others. The disagreements will be fought out rather than walked away from, and the ones that can't be settled will be lived with.

What *Is* a Family, Anyway?

How realistic is it to think that disagreements among family members can be worked out in the way we're suggesting? Doubts about the possibility of familial teamwork are magnified by the popular idea that the family has somehow "dissolved." With divorce so prevalent, a big increase in the number of parents raising children by themselves, people living together without marriage, same-sex couples, and spousal or parental abuse so widely reported, isn't the kind of family we're talking about here—tight-knit, with everybody concerned about one another—an endangered species?

In our opinion, the family as an institution is pretty tough. It's been around since prehistoric times, which is reason enough to suppose it will last a few more years. But the form itself has altered over time—an alteration that in our part of the world has lately accelerated. It's this shape-shifting that gives rise to confusion, fear, and distrust. What does it mean to be a family nowadays? Who's out, who's in, and what follows from being in or out?

Our first idea is that families aren't defined so much by what kind of people they're made up of, as by what kind of work goes on in them. Despite what Webster's dictionary might say, not all families are "a group of individuals living under one roof and usually under one head," or "the basic unit in society having as its nucleus two or more adults living together and cooperating in care and rearing of their own or adopted children." Lots of people regard themselves as family despite the fact that they are not sharing the same residence, don't recognize anyone in particular as a "head," and are no longer (if they ever were) involved in the task of raising kids. Why do they regard themselves as family? We suggest it's because of the special jobs that are going on within their relationships.

Families—both the kinds people think of as normal and the more offbeat varieties—are places where people get a kind of intimacy that is extremely important to being socially, emotionally, and morally whole. The ongoing, committed, and long-standing relationships found in families allow them to mirror back to us a detailed and historically informed knowledge of who we are. In fact, the members of our family have a great deal to do with *making* us who we are.

Even if you can't stand your sister, then, the fact that you and she go way back and were raised inside an intimate relationship means that she's an important part of your life story. She may have drifted away in adulthood; maybe for one bitter reason or another there's no relationship left between you. But if the two of you now have a responsibility to look after a parent who is suffering from dementia (because you got the good of being loved by that parent when you were children), then it will be up to you both to rebuild your own relationship, at least to the degree that allows you to cooperate in the care of your parent. In other words, being out of the family doesn't always mean you get to stay out.

What if the person who's out of the family is the person who needs the care? Suppose, for example, she is an alcoholic mother who was at best unreliable when her son was little and now that he's grown is often abusive. Does he have a duty to stay in a loving relationship with her? Relationships take at least two people, so to the extent that the alcoholism has broken this one down, there's little the son can do about it. He certainly doesn't have the full range of duties to his mother that Janet has to hers, although if there's no one else to make arrangements for her care, common decency requires him to do it. He shouldn't allow her needs to jeopardize the well-being of his own household, but those needs do pull her a little farther back into his family.

Despite all the frictions and failures in families, people still need their connections. If people are important, then these attachments are important as well, and worth the trouble it takes to maintain them.

DOING THE FAMILY HUDDLE

Since there are good reasons for Janet, Pam, and Nicholas to work hard at staying on good terms and cooperating in their mother's care, they'll have to keep talking to one another. What might these talks be like, and what can and can't they accomplish? In outline, the idea of Dwayne Bailey's "Family Huddle" is very simple. The members of the family share concerns, pool ideas, make and revise plans, and provide support for one another. Ideally, some of these meetings are face to face, and include the person who is ill. If she is only mildly demented, she may have lost her ability to initiate long-term planning while still being capable of discussing her concerns, hopes, fears, and wishes. Such discussion would give the family useful guidance for future decision making, both in situations where a particular problem has been anticipated and in those where it hasn't. Even when something unexpected comes up, if family members have thoroughly explored things with the ill person, they may be in a better position to understand what she would say about the matter at hand if she were able.

Other family huddles needn't include the ill person, and needn't have everybody in the same room. Whether over the phone or through some medium like e-mail, such conversations can provide the rest of the family with an opportunity to express their views without censoring themselves for the ill person's benefit. They give people a chance to say what they are prepared to do and what they are not prepared to do. Over time, as the full dimensions of the problem become plainer, such talks make it easier to see whether people's assessments are realistic, fair to themselves, and fair to others. This in turn allows the family to rearrange the division of labor.

How spouses, siblings, and adult children respond to the earliest stages of the dementia may take on a special significance that goes beyond that moment. The way the first decisions are made, conflicts resolved, and problems met, and the way the family initially comes to think and feel about the person who is ill can set patterns for what is to come.

A big task for the family at this point will be figuring out the best ways to share the responsibilities. Families so often simply expect that one member—usually a woman—will be the primary caretaker. The others then take less active roles, deciding for themselves, privately, how much or how little they're going to do. This is a good way to breed resentment, ill will, and defensiveness. While in practice it's highly unlikely that tasks can always be divided equally among family members, determining just what would count as fair and what people can appropriately expect of one another is a chore that needs to be undertaken early on.

What the O'Keefes, for example, worked out was that Ms. O'Keefe and Janet would continue to live together, and Janet would do most of the day-to-day helping out. This arrangement was to continue for one year—the amount of time Janet felt she'd need to make serious plans about her own further education and career. During that period, her siblings would provide regular breaks for her. After that time, the whole situation would be reevaluated. If it turned out for the best that Janet continue to live with her mother, the others would consider themselves obliged to help her financially, perhaps contributing to her tuition or staking her to a start in business. Or maybe it would be necessary for Pam and Nicholas to help pay for a full-time caregiver.

Anyone who wants to remain in an ongoing, familial relationship, no matter how distant, with a person suffering from dementia will have to come to terms with the full impact of the disease. We've already explored the special reason why Janet, Pam, and Nicholas need to do this. But what about other family members? What about Nicholas's wife, and Pam's less-than-perfect husband? If these people wish to continue in a familial relationship with the ones caring for Ms. O'Keefe, they too have to become part of the process of providing care.

One of the reasons for this is simple fairness—to the relationship with Ms. O'Keefe, as well as to the relationships with their own spouses and with Janet. Any relationship with another person that is more than simply a matter of using her involves some readiness to take the other person's point of view seriously, on that person's own terms. If one member of the family is doing most of the hands-on work, other family members who wish to maintain a relationship with her will have to look at the situation from her perspective and respond accordingly. If they think she is doing more than is necessary, or that she exaggerates the importance of what she is doing, taking her seriously means talking things over with her to see if some agreement can be reached.

Family huddles give people a chance to explore their fears and hopes, weave a little extra solidarity into the web of family life, and carve up the tasks of caregiving. They also have a fourth function—one so important we're going to devote the next chapter to it. It's the function of visualizing the future of the person with the dementing illness—a process called *advance planning*. What people do in the future to respond to the illness will have a greater effect on the ill person than on anyone else involved. For that reason, the person should be encouraged to participate in planning that future while she can still help determine what it will be.

When the Family's Response Is Less Than Admirable

Ms. O'Keefe hates to think about the future, but she knows her children are working hard to help her and she wants to make things easier for them. So she did her best in the two face-to-face conversations Nicholas and Pam were able to attend. The monthly conference calls that followed the face-to-face visits were a big help to Janet, because they made her feel she wasn't having to cope with her mother's illness all by herself. As the months wore on, however, Janet began to get the distinct impression that what she'd feared earlier was indeed coming true: Nicholas and Pam were going to leave her holding the baby. Well before the year was over, there was one "good" reason after another why they had to cancel the weekends with their mother that would give Janet the breaks they'd all agreed she should have. They started talking about the possibility of a full-time caregiver, but hinted that it would be up to Janet to arrange it without any help from them. And any time she's reported to them how tired she is, or how Mom's behavior is worrying her, instead of offering sympathy and support, they've made it clear they think she should put Mom in a nursing home. But Janet doesn't agree. She sees that her mom loves her own home and feels safest there, and thinks she's perfectly capable of living there for quite a while so long as there's someone looking after her.

Let's suppose that Janet is right about this, and that Pam and Nicholas aren't living up to their responsibilities. Let's say that they are, in fact, letting everybody down. When Janet pointed this out to them, they didn't mend their ways; instead, they simply came up with fresh excuses. So it seems that Janet can't make them love their mother better, or force them to treat Janet fairly, or get them to do what's right. It looks like she's stuck.

And so she is. But she's stuck because she's remaining loyal to her mother and to her own moral commitments. In keeping faith with her mother by trying to respond lovingly and imaginatively to her illness, Janet is also keeping faith with herself. She is exercising the personal integrity that allows her mother to depend on her, and in doing so she is becoming more like the person she would ideally like to be. She is deriving quiet satisfaction from living well with herself. From that point of view, she's not so much stuck as standing fast.

Moreover, after doing everything she could to involve her brother and sister in their mother's care, Janet had the grace to stop hammering at a door that wasn't going to open. She acknowledged the limits of Nicholas's and Pam's loyalties and didn't waste valuable energy in trying to make them be other than who they were. Nor did she waste energy in dwelling on her grievances. Her opinion of her brother and sister has been lowered, but she's trying to remember that they may have difficulties she knows nothing about, and countless other calls on their time and attention.

Reacting so calmly to a situation that can be very hard for a very long time requires a clear-sightedness that's bound to desert Janet on occasion. This ability to see both what can and what can't be done, and to see where some of her own limits lie, has been the source of the grace and integrity with which she meets her mother's needs. There will be times, however, when her moral vision will fail her—when she loses her sense of humor and gets things out of proportion, when she doesn't see her mother with the eye of loving attention. But she's worked out what her overall goal has to be, and we don't think she'll lose sight of it for long: to welcome into her own life the project of looking after her mother as well as she can.

2

Making Plans
for the Future

WHEN JOSHUA CANTOR turned seventy, he lost two of the most important things in his life. One loss, the jewelry business to which he had devoted nearly forty years, was expected and regretfully planned for. It was past time to sell. Running the business had become an uphill battle against the large jewelry store chains, and profits had dropped off in the past several years even though Joshua had been putting in longer hours than when the place was in its prime. Besides, he was tired and getting on in years—he didn't need all the worry and responsibility.

The other loss was a shock. His wife, to whom he'd been happily married since he was twenty-five, died suddenly of a heart attack. She was a few years younger than he and had been so healthy and active all her life that he had always assumed she would outlive him. It wasn't until after she died that he realized how heavily he'd depended on her. Her unexpected passing shook him deeply, unseating all his hopes for a peaceful and rewarding retirement.

Mr. Cantor is now seventy-three and dealing with yet another blow. Since shortly after his wife's death, he had seemed to his family and friends somehow less able to cope with life, more absentminded, more easily confused. His children chalked up these lapses to the natural forces of grief and adjustment to widowerhood, but they also urged him to see his doctor. The doctor's examination led to repeated visits and those visits to very bad news: Mr. Cantor has Alzheimer's disease.

Like Ms. O'Keefe, Mr. Cantor and his children struggled to acknowledge and do something about the situation into which they had been thrust. Unlike the O'Keefes, however, they made good-faith efforts at first to work together as a family and try to sort out what to do. But now that Mr. Cantor and his family are starting to emerge from the shock and to confront the question of how to share the rest of their life together, a serious difference of opinion has arisen.

John, Mr. Cantor's eldest son, wants his father to transfer his assets to John's sister Anne immediately. Sheltering this money with Anne, John feels, is much better than letting a nursing home eat it up at the rate of sixty thousand dollars or more a year.

Medicare won't pay for nursing home care, but Medicaid will—as long as Mr. Cantor can prove that he owns nothing more than his house, his car, personal possessions, and a modest amount of cash. John thinks they'll have to act fast, since, to avoid penalties, the money has to have been transferred three years before a person applies for Medicaid. There's no telling how much longer Mr. Cantor will be capable of making the transfer, and no telling when he may need daily professional care.

John points out that his dad's assets aren't just money—they represent the full forty years of his life's work. It's only right that the family should do what it can to preserve that, especially since sheltering the money with Anne is perfectly legal.

"Look," he says to his dad. "The whole health care system's badly designed and unfair to people like you. It's built around high-tech, intensive, short-term treatments that are supposed to make a sick person well. It's *not* designed for people with long-term problems like Alzheimer's disease, who need lower-tech care—but for months or years—and who aren't ever going to get well. People like you get nothing while somebody who needs his second round of triple coronary bypass surgery gets a full ride. It's crazy. Why should somebody with a heart condition be covered and treated better than you? You're being discriminated against."

John is arguing as if the problem is to try, in the

face of an unresponsive and unjust social system, to pull what his father has worked for all his life out of the wreck of the disease that is slowly destroying him. While John doesn't say so out loud, he also thinks that in his best moments his father surely wouldn't want to spend all that money— money that could go to his children and his children's children—just to keep a badly demented person in a nicer nursing home for a few more months. If they help their dad stay at home until he's past caring about the amenities and then let Medicaid kick in, he'll get adequate care and they'll all have saved the money he had worked so hard to accumulate.

Mr. Cantor is, as he puts it, underwhelmed by John's plan. So is Anne, for two reasons. For one, she's afraid that if she accepts the transfer, she's also accepting John's share of the responsibility for her father's care. Anne has a little girl, a husband she's quite fond of, a room full of kindergartners she loves to teach, and she wouldn't at all mind becoming pregnant again. While she realizes that a good deal of her father's care will fall to her, she's determined that it will be a fair amount, one that she can balance with her other responsibilities. She's carefully watching all of John's moves in this discussion, afraid of the many good reasons he'll come up with for not doing too much to look after his father.

Like her brother, Anne thinks things that she

doesn't say out loud—not even to herself. In the back of her mind, though, she wonders whether John won't duck out on her when their dad's situation gets really bad. For most purposes John's pretty reliable—he came in very handy when Anne was a teenager and needed her old car fixed, for example. What's not so clear is whether he can stay involved and available for what might be years as their dad gets progressively worse and taking care of him gets progressively harder. John's a little bit like the health care system he's so busy criticizing: good for acute problems, not so hot for long-term care.

Anne also can't shake the feeling that this asset-transfer scheme is really nothing less than a move to defraud the government—which is to say, the taxpayers—since Medicaid was never designed for middle-class people. Her brother disagrees.

"I'm telling you, this is perfectly legal," he insists. "My lawyer says there's a whole new specialty called elder law that's grown up around this problem. It's got its own professional society— the Academy of Elder Law Attorneys—and somewhere around four thousand members nationwide. It's a field that didn't even exist ten years ago, but it's growing because health care costs are growing and the number of old people in this country is growing, and people are having to figure out how to deal with what's basically a new trend. Nobody's talking about breaking the law. What I'm proposing is legal."

"Okay, it's legal," Anne says, jangling her turquoise and silver bracelets irritably. "That doesn't make it ethical. The rules about who's eligible for Medicaid were made through a democratic process, don't forget, and they weren't made with this little end-run in mind. Before Pop got sick, you never had any problem with the idea that Medicaid was supposed to be available for poor people, not for people like us. If you gave it any thought at all, you were probably just thankful that your taxes weren't any higher."

"As a matter of fact, I didn't think about it. But now that I have, I honestly don't see that Pop has some kind of patriotic duty to save all his money over the next several years, just so he'll have it available to pay for a nursing home he'll probably never need."

John gets up from the sofa and goes to kneel by his father's chair. "Look, Pop. Suppose you decided tomorrow that you wanted to take a trip to Israel—to see Jerusalem again one more time while you've still got your health. You know what we'd say? We'd say, Fine, do it. Go to Jerusalem, have a good time. Maybe that's what you *do* want to do. If it is, I'm all for it. So's Anne. And if it's not immoral for you to transfer your assets to El Al, it's not immoral for you to transfer them to Anne."

On thinking it over, Anne admits that there might be something to this way of looking at it, but she's not as confident about this as John is. For one thing, transferring the money from her father to herself will make it easier to put Pop into a nursing home sooner rather than later. She's uncomfortable about this. If the only way the family can preserve his estate is to keep him at home as long as possible, then that's an incentive to keep him there, even if it means considerable extra trouble for his children and their families. On the other hand, if they already have the whole estate, then there's only Pop's own well-being to consider, and there won't be any reason to give that any more weight than the interests of other family members. Pop suddenly becomes just another contender for the family's resources. Anne doesn't particularly like the fact that she's thinking in these terms, but she is.

Mr. Cantor is "underwhelmed" for another reason. He's not much worried about whether John will be involved in his day-to-day care—he takes it for granted that he won't be. Nor is he worried about the Medicaid question. He's been a scrupulous taxpayer all his life, and the only feeling he has about the government is that it's finally time for him to get something back from it. No, what troubles Mr. Cantor is that giving up control of his assets makes him feel as though he's giving up control over himself, not to mention cutting the ties to his past. He feels as if he's cooperating with, rather than fighting, what the disease is doing to him.

<small>MAKING PLANS TOGETHER: UP CLOSE AND PERSONAL</small>

This family obviously faces a number of problems, some on the surface, some buried deeper. They're disagreeing about who owes what to whom, they don't completely trust each other, and Anne in particular isn't altogether sure she trusts herself. How can good solutions to the moral problems of caregiving emerge among people so divided?

Part of the trouble here is that the Cantors all have different ideas about how we should live—about what makes life good and what should matter to us, both on a daily basis and in the larger scheme of things. Anne and John don't agree, for example, on what a good son or daughter should be willing to do for a parent, or what a good father should want to give his children, or what good citizens owe to their community or country. They also have different assumptions about whether being a woman automatically means you should be the caregiver, and different hopes and expectations about their own futures. Some of these differences seem to be colliding at breakneck speed.

But different ideas about how we should live often go along with other kinds of differences. We see the effect of the Cantor children's different personalities: Anne is an intense, romantic person who dresses flamboyantly, and John is more businesslike and dispassionate. Such different personal styles can raise suspicions about whether everyone is really acting in good faith. Fiscal conservatism can look, to a romantic, like greed; emotional intensity, to a reserved person, can look like unreliability. Furthermore, Anne and John give different accounts of their history as children growing up together. These differences can be the basis of disagreements, sometimes nasty ones, among family members.

Why Is Advance Planning a Good Idea?

Advance planning might seem to run contrary to the old proverb, "Don't trouble trouble till trouble troubles you." Having disturbing talks with your relatives about difficult possibilities that *might* crop up at some time in the future sounds like a painful and pointless way to spend your time—something like arguing with your ex-spouse. Still, we think there are three good reasons for the Cantors to try to do some advance planning together.

The first reason has to do with Joshua Cantor himself. One of the most important ways competent, mature individuals express their personhood is by making their own decisions about how they will try to lead their lives. Mr. Cantor's situation has suddenly changed, and he hasn't had time to figure out how best to be himself in these new circumstances. In the process of thinking about what the disease is likely to do to him, getting a sense of the difficult decisions that have to be made, and making as many as possible while he is still able, he can examine, refine, and expand his own particular view of what the good life is for him. For many people, decisions about how to live out the last chapters of their lives present the final opportunity to tie up loose ends and to affirm the important values they have lived by. Creating opportunities for someone to have a say in these matters, even when he is ill with a dementing disease, is a way of respecting that person's dignity. It's also a way of resisting a major temptation: to treat the person as if he were a child.

Anne's in favor of discussing Pop's future with Pop. Assuming too quickly that he's too confused to do certain things may actually make him unable to do them, she thinks. And if making decisions is a way for him to express who he is, well, she wants to do right by him. She doesn't want to contribute to any sense that Pop has been demoted from his status as a dignified adult. Of course, she doesn't know for a fact that he'll be interested in making plans with her and John about his illness. However, he used to take the lead in things like helping the kids choose what college to go to or planning the family's vacations, so Anne thinks that involving him in their decision making is an expression of respect that's appropriate for him. It wouldn't have mattered as much for her mom, who never thought of herself as the person in charge of decisions. But Pop did.

The second reason why at least some advance planning should take place with everybody together—this is John's reason—is that since he and Anne are going to have to call the shots later on, they have a responsibility to try to learn what their dad needs and wants. John doesn't think it would be right to step up his dad's care when he's dying, for example, if it turns out that Pop would've hated that—and especially if he had never bothered to ask. Just as important, he thinks, is making sure that Pop knows what he and Anne are willing to go along with. For instance, if Pop thinks he's going to keep living by himself until he's bedridden, and the kids think he'll have to have supervision long before that, he needs to know that they won't honor his wish. Then they may be able to come up with a plan they all can live with.

While not all problems will be solved nor all disagreements headed off (talking about things in the open can sometimes lead to even sharper disagreements), much of the friction between patient and caregiver stems from different beliefs about what is actually happening. If agreement can be reached about that, then it can more easily be reached about what should be done in response, and about who should do it. In any case, it's worth clearing up misunderstandings based on assumptions that seem obvious to one person, but not at all obvious to anyone else.

A third, often unappreciated reason for advance planning is that people don't always *have* clear preferences about things that may be completely foreign to them. The Cantors have no previous experience with Alzheimer's disease. Do *you* know what medical treatment you'd want if at some point you were demented and in a diaper and living in a nursing home, and you came down with a life-threatening pneumonia? Most of us don't have a fully formed preference about something like that, because we don't know enough about what it would be like for us, or what the fallout would be for other people. Figuring out what we would want later on is often best done in dialogue with other concerned and involved people—the more so, as those people will surely be affected by what we want.

Why Is Advance Planning Dangerous?

"I'll tell you what makes me so nervous about talking with Pop and John about Pop's care," Anne said on the phone to a friend one day. "I'm afraid that if we disagree with each other, people's feelings will be hurt, and we might even end up on bad terms with each other."

"Well," said the friend, "at my office, people disagree with each other all the time and everything jogs along pretty smoothly anyway."

"Yeah, but that's because when you're at work you don't really care if you step on a few toes here and there. When it's your brother and you love him, you can't help caring."

"True," her friend agreed. "And your family stays in your life longer than your co-workers do. My sister is always my sister, even when she's being awful, whereas my boss is my boss only until I quit—or get fired—and go to work for someone else."

This special feature of family relationships has moral implications. You might not be willing to say what you honestly think to your brother, either because you don't want to hurt his feelings, or because you think you have to paper over your differences with him so there won't be a visible rupture in the family. This is what's going on between Anne and John. Anne is uneasy about her brother's real commitment to the project they're trying to put together. She worries that if she pushes too hard against his point of view, he may simply become disaffected, both with her and with the task of caring for Pop.

John, on the other hand, has implicit confidence in Anne's commitment; he knows that she's in it for the long haul, that she'll always be there for him when he wants her, and always be there for

his dad as well. This doesn't mean that he's plotting to exploit her; fairness is a value for him, just as it is for her. It does mean that he's more comfortable with arguing vigorously for his own perspective on things. He doesn't want to hurt her feelings, of course, but he thinks that the issues they are considering are of great importance, and worth some hurt feelings if necessary. He doesn't worry that any real damage will be done.

These differences are impossible to set completely to one side. Family history, clashing moral perspectives, personal idiosyncracies, and gender stereotypes may all play a role here, and are deep and powerful forces. They can be kept from disrupting the proceedings, however, if the involved parties have a clear sense up front of what they're trying to do and of what might get in the way.

ADVANCE PLANNING: HOW TO BEGIN

"I don't understand why you're pushing this," said Anne to John the next time they stopped by Pop's house together. "I definitely don't want to take over the responsibility for handling Pop's money." She was perched on the arm of her dad's chair, and now she reached over and rumpled his hair. "I don't see the point in it, Pop. If you ever need more care than we can give you, well, John and I will work something out. Together. We'll hire somebody, or try to get creative about involving

other people. Maybe we'll reach a point where you run out of money and need us to help pay your bills, but we can cross that bridge when we come to it."

"Yeah, but the time is going to come when we have to take more responsibility for you, Pop," John replied. "Not right away, of course—I don't mean that. And naturally, whatever we have to do, we'll do it together. I'm just saying that now is the time we should be protecting Pop's assets."

John tapped the table with his pen. "The best way to do that is to have him live here as long as he can and then have him move in with one of us. Either way, we'll keep him at home as long as it matters to him to be at home. We won't move you to a nursing home, Pop. Not unless you get to where you don't really care where you are—and that might never happen. But if it ever did, at least you'd have the comfort of knowing that your property is safe."

At this point, Mr. Cantor rose to his feet and left the room, shutting the door hard.

Whatever else they disagreed about, Anne and John were of one mind in seeing this as a bad start. They decided to put the money issue on the back burner for a while and start over again. Advance planning still seemed like a good idea, but they were going to have to go at it more thoughtfully.

They began by proposing that their discussions

be fairly formal. The family would set aside regular times to talk over how things were going with Mr. Cantor's illness, what needed to be done next, and what would need attention in the future. Topics unrelated to his disease wouldn't be discussed during the times set aside for Mr. Cantor.

John thought it would be a good idea to write up what happened at each meeting and to make copies for everyone. This was partly so they could keep track of what had been decided, but also to later convince doctors and other caregivers outside the family that their decisions had something of Mr. Cantor's own authority behind them. Anne agreed, so long as John was willing to rotate the note-taking task, rather than sticking her with it permanently.

Anne and John also tried to figure out who needed to be in on these discussions and who could safely be left out. Mr. Cantor did have a younger brother in California, but their lives hadn't been closely connected for a long time, and Mr. Cantor thought that just keeping George informed of what was happening would probably be enough. Furthermore, he was adamant about not involving any of his friends in these discussions. So the meetings would be held with Anne and her husband Philip, John and his wife Wendy, and John and Wendy's two teenage sons, who were close to their grandfather. That way, no one who needed to be in was left out; no one who wanted out was forced in. Other families may not, of course, be quite so lucky in these respects.

Another important point that Anne and John agreed on was that, while advance planning was a good idea, it would be impossible to foresee everything that might affect their sense of what was best, or even feasible. Their plans might have to be revised at a later date, and if they paid attention to the *reasons* behind the decisions they made now, they'd be that much better able to preserve the spirit of those decisions in the future. Therefore, the reasons would be written down along with the decisions.

Anne and John also thought about how to make the conferences hospitable enough so that people would feel they could say what they really thought. They reminded each other up front that the problem of their father's illness was a problem that everyone in the family had agreed to share equally. They acknowledged that personality differences would get in the way of complete openness and equality in their discussions, and they all agreed to try to compensate for this.

So that was the plan: Mr. Cantor and his family caregivers would meet together regularly to discuss how people were doing, to identify issues, to make new plans, and to revisit old ones. Mr. Cantor would be a part of these discussions for as long as he could. But even after he was no longer able to participate meaningfully, the family would continue to meet.

As often happens, however, the reality turned out to be a little different from the plan.

Advance Planning: Can We Talk?

Advance planning sessions are supposed to help the person with the dementing illness get a sense of what decisions may need to be made and what the options are, and then to actually make some choices. Many of the choices have to do with what will happen in the future, when a person like Mr. Cantor won't be able to fully understand what's going on and what might be done about it. Some of these situations can be forecast fairly well and the planning sessions are an opportunity to do that.

Mr. Cantor had already given some thought to this sort of thing. After his wife's death, he filed a legal document called a health care proxy, which is also known as a durable power of attorney for health care decisions. This document is one form of advance directive; it appoints someone to make decisions about treatment you will or will not get, in the event that you are too ill to make these decisions for yourself. Health care proxies allow you to choose someone who will make the decisions in your place.

Other advance directives—living wills, or, more

broadly, treatment directives—contain directions not about *who* decides but about *what* decisions should be made. For instance, a person may direct that if he ever is so unfortunate as to fall into an irreversible coma, he doesn't want to be kept alive on a respirator. Or he might direct that if he is dying of an incurable cancer, he wants only comfort care. Of course, it's also possible to have "mixed" advance directives, which both name a person to make decisions and give that person specific directions about the patient's health care preferences.

In some states—like New York—living wills haven't been recognized by the legislature (which doesn't mean they wouldn't be honored in court), but people are encouraged to name a "health care agent" who will make medical decisions for them should it become necessary. The agent's power isn't unlimited, and depending where you live, there may be rather strict laws about it. For example, if you don't want to have artificially provided food and fluids under certain conditions, in some states you have to give your agent specific authorization to refuse that treatment.

Three years ago Mr. Cantor executed an advance directive in which he named his son as his agent for health care and specifically gave him authorization to make decisions about tube-feedings. However, at that time, he and John didn't really discuss what Mr. Cantor might want under various circumstances. Today, John realizes that the time to talk about it is now. If they don't, John may come to find himself in a very uncomfortable position, because he'll be expected to speak on his dad's behalf without really knowing what Mr. Cantor had in mind.

But here the Cantors ran into yet another snag. Although Mr. Cantor is perfectly capable of deciding whether he still wants John to be his health care agent, he's having considerable difficulty with his short-term memory. He forgets that he's ill with Alzheimer's disease. As a result, he's not particularly motivated to talk about his future. The whole idea leaves him cold. He hates the prospect of being so sick that other people have to do his thinking for him, and he didn't much enjoy what happened the first time John and Anne sat down to talk with him. His reluctance may also have something to do with the idea that his kids already know or should be able to figure out what he would want. Isn't that how he raised them—to take care of him in his old age and not bother him with questions?

Here, John and Anne confront what is clearly another moral problem. Should they respect their father's unwillingness to discuss the future—which would mean, of course, that they will be on their own when hard decisions need to be made? Or is it, rather, the part of a loving and judicious family to take an active role in starting the discussion?

Shouldn't they *insist* that their father pay attention to the decisions that are at hand, and do his best to give directions about them?

The answer depends on just how unwilling he is. Making good decisions for a confused person is not a trivial problem, and the burdens imposed upon the proxy decision makers are not light. In most situations similar to the one Mr. Cantor's children find themselves in, it would be both irresponsible and imprudent for the children simply to take the path of least resistance and not raise any questions at all. On the other hand, if Mr. Cantor firmly and repeatedly refuses to talk about the future, it might mean he wishes that his children would simply lift the burden of choice from his shoulders. He might be signaling that he trusts them to deal responsibly with issues he would very much rather not face himself.

There is another, even more complicated possibility. The children might be able to persuade Mr. Cantor to discuss his future, but at great cost to himself. He might be deeply disturbed and frightened by these conversations, and at a loss to understand why he is being asked to do something so intensely disagreeable. The thought of this possibility put a considerable weight on Anne and John for a time. They had to decide whether to push their father to tell them what he thought, and if they did push, how hard. They had to determine what they'd do if he continued to be unwilling to participate in planning discussions.

Anne grew so frustrated during this time that when she stopped by John's house one Saturday afternoon, it was either vent her feelings or burst. "How on earth can Pop expect us to steer blindfolded? Dammit, he has no *right* to saddle us with all the decisions that'll have to be made for him over the next few years when we have no idea what he would have wanted. We're just supposed to guess? What if we guess wrong? Honest to God, I have never seen anybody so pigheaded and downright *selfish* in all my life!"

Her sister-in-law handed her a Diet Coke while her brother propped himself against the kitchen counter, arms folded across his chest, grinning. "Getting on your wick, isn't he, Annie? I haven't seen you blow into the house like this since I let your boom box fall into the swimming pool when we were in high school. I think you're being too hard on the old man. I mean, Pop's got a *right* to make decisions about his own life, but I don't think that means he's got a *duty* to make 'em—especially since we're around to do it for him. Besides, I'm not so sure he *can* make 'em." He turned to his wife. "I didn't have a chance to tell you this yet, Wendy, but when I took Pop to the hardware store this morning he suddenly looked at me and said, 'You know, you're my favorite customer.' I said, 'Pop, I'm your son!' So he said, 'Oh well, that explains it, then.' It was all I could do not to laugh out loud."

Mr. Cantor remained reluctant to take an active role in planning his future, so his children finally regrouped. Although they felt rather peculiar about meeting without him, John, Wendy, and their two teenage boys did get together at Anne and Philip's house to discuss the situation. They decided there was no good reason to change the arrangement that had been made three years ago: John would continue to be the official proxy decision maker for his dad. But John wanted other family members—particularly his sister—to be involved in the decision making. He didn't want to do it all by himself if he didn't have to, and he also wanted to start deciding things right away. Just as he was strongly of the opinion that his dad's financial situation had to be dealt with immediately, so too he felt it was crucial that they imagine what medical and familial problems might come up, and at least sketch out potential solutions.

Anne thought it wasn't enough to anticipate problems and develop strategies on their own. She thought they also ought to let their dad know what they came up with so he could veto a decision if he wanted to. She pointed out that there was a difference between having to be involved in thinking through lots of complicated alternatives, on the one hand, and simply agreeing to or rejecting a scheme on the other. Just because Pop wouldn't participate in planning didn't mean he wouldn't want to know what they had worked out for him, or wouldn't appreciate the chance to object. At least, she argued, they should give him the opportunity to respond. And anyway, it was always possible that if they presented him with some sketched-out plans, Mr. Cantor might be willing to fill in the details himself.

John wondered if going back to him with their ideas wouldn't be hard on the old man. "Why shove possibilities down his throat when it's clear he doesn't want to deal with them? It seems to me he's already at the point where any kind of planning or organization overwhelms him, and what we're talking about here isn't just complicated, it's nasty and unpleasant. We can handle it without involving him. We lived with him long enough to know how he feels."

"Sure we did," Anne snorted. "We lived with Mom for a long time too, and we couldn't even buy her the kind of clothes she liked. Remember that suede skirt we got her for her birthday one year, and how she wore it all that day and then left it hanging in the closet? Remember how bad we felt because we'd guessed wrong? Well, what we have to guess about here is going to make us feel a whole lot worse if we don't have some sense that we're doing what he wants."

This struck Wendy, the boys, and Anne's husband Philip as a fair point, and, after some discussion, John agreed that he and his sister would let Pop know what they'd been talking about. So Anne and John did have some talks with Mr. Cantor about what they felt should be done. In the course of these talks, the older man seemed to become a little more comfortable with the subject, and responded to some of their proposals and opinions. Over time, they had the chance to talk about—and write down—his thoughts about many important things: that he didn't care so much about driving his car, for example, but he was damned if he would give up carpentry even if there was a chance he might hurt himself. And that he expected them to keep him out of the nursing home, but he also didn't want to be a burden to them. Anne toyed with the idea of taping these discussions, thinking that maybe having a record of *how* Pop said something would sometimes be as useful as a record of *what* he said. But, like a lot of interesting ideas, that one fell through the cracks.

Mr. Cantor's concerns about being a burden to them were the first things they talked about. These were followed by issues of privacy and contact with others. Like Ms. O'Keefe, Mr. Cantor had been a rather private person, but he did have several close friends. He both very much wanted to see them and very much wanted to avoid them. With the encouragement of his kids, Mr. Cantor eventually came to hope that one or two of his closest friends might be invited back into his life, and that they might even help him out with a few things that were getting beyond him.

There were many other topics the group eventually touched on. When he couldn't live by himself anymore, would he rather move in with Anne or have a home health aide? Would he like to get to know something about the activity groups and special classes that were available for people with Alzheimer's disease? Would he care to visit some local nursing homes to see if they were better than he thought?

Questions about medical care were more difficult. The family wanted to know what they should do if other medical problems came up. Having Alzheimer's doesn't, after all, protect a person from heart attacks, strokes, or cancer. If Mr. Cantor should become seriously ill, or badly injured, would he want to undergo intensive care, or would he rather just be kept comfortable, even if that meant he would die sooner? How about the kinds of medical treatment he might require because of the Alzheimer's disease itself? What did he think about being fed through a tube if the dementia progressed to the point where he couldn't eat anymore?

And then there was John's pet problem: what should be done about Mr. Cantor's money? This was very much tangled up with the question of nursing home care. Of course Mr. Cantor never wanted to go to a nursing home, but what if they just couldn't manage to take care of him themselves? What if he started wandering away from home and getting lost, or keeping everybody up all night, or hitting and yelling at people? He might be willing to have his children run his errands, keep his checkbook balanced, dress him, and make sure he took his pills, but how would he feel about one of them bathing him? Giving him a bedpan? Spoon-feeding him? Massaging him to prevent bedsores? Changing his diaper?

Ethical Decision Making: More Than Preferences

While people don't always agree about how to make good moral decisions, nobody thinks you can do it with bad information. Anne, John, Wendy, Philip, and the boys, then, needed to do more than figure out whether and how to involve Mr. Cantor in their advance planning conferences. They also had to figure out what needed to be decided in these conferences. And to do that, they had to gather a fair amount of information. This is not an easy task, because services for the aged and for dementia sufferers are scattered; there's no central clearinghouse. So both children had to put in long and sometimes frustrating sessions on the telephone.

Anne, John, and their families had an even harder job as well. They had to figure out how to put together a fair and reasonable strategy for caring in the light of the many different needs that confronted them. Like almost everybody else, they believe that fairness is as important a part of good moral decision making as is good information, but agreeing on what's fair in a particular case is often very difficult.

This was another job that couldn't be done without better information about what kinds of help their father was likely to need over time, and what kinds of help were actually available. Some of this information came from his doctor, some from the Alzheimer's Association, and some from books. Some also came from the planning conferences themselves, as each learned more about the others' situations, and looked for ways to fit new challenges as comfortably as possible into their established ways of living. They discovered that a fair amount of the information they needed was readily at hand, in themselves and their own lives, in what they valued, and in what mattered most to those they loved. Weighing all this information allowed them to get a better sense of what was possible if they were to help their father and still keep faith with their other responsibilities and commitments.

One effect of their early discussions was that John stopped insisting on having the money question settled his way. He could see that not everyone was willing to fall into line with his plan—that in fact, money was a very divisive topic. Rather than get bogged down in disagreement, he realized that it would be a good idea to see what financial issues they could agree on before they started on the controversies.

Anne consulted a lawyer to help with the financial part of her father's advance planning, and got a very careful explanation of what their legal options were. In the end, they decided that his money should be used mainly to provide for his care and comfort. Here's how they reasoned.

"It'll save trouble all the way around if Pop gives one of us power of attorney now," said Anne to John over the phone. "Otherwise, when he's really out of it and we have to pay bills or sell his house or whatever, we'll have to go to court and that's time-consuming, not to mention expensive. I think he'd be willing to let one of us *handle* his money, so long as he feels that nobody's trying to take it away from him."

"Of course nobody's trying to take it away from him. I was trying to shelter it so that nobody *could* take it away from him. I've been saying all along that he should be calling the shots here. It's his money. Absolutely. He has a perfect right to do anything he wants with it."

"Right. And our job is to try to figure out what that is, because he doesn't want to talk about it. You know, this would be a lot simpler if we could just lift up the top of his head and see what preferences he's carrying around in there. Because, as you say, we're only supposed to make sure that the money's used the way he'd prefer, without—"

"What?"

Anne was silent for a moment. "Well, I was going to say without considering anything or anybody else. But I wonder if I believe that. I mean, maybe it's not just Pop's preferences, but Pop himself—all of him—we're supposed to think about when we have to decide things for him."

"What do you mean?"

"Well, I was thinking about what we'd do if Pop's mind was just fine and he decided to spend all his money at the races or on a luxury cruise, even though he knew you needed it desperately and had never asked him for any kind of loan before. I think I'd argue with him. I'd tell him he'd always been too good a person to suddenly stop caring about the people who love him and need him. I'd tell him he couldn't do what he wanted just because he felt like it, and he ought to care about doing what's right."

"Okay. That's nice. So?"

"So, he'd agree with me. That's how he brought us up, for heaven's sake. So how come now that we have to make decisions for him, we're suddenly changing the rules and considering only what he might like for himself? Why aren't we also thinking about his commitments to things like justice and honesty, courage, compassion for people, kindness, how much he loves us? I guess I think if we're really looking after him right, we have to care about those things for him too."

John and Anne talked this idea over for a while and came to believe that, within limits, anyway, they did want to consider how their decisions on their dad's behalf fit within these broader moral commitments. Coming back to the question of how to manage their dad's money, they asked themselves whether anyone would be treated unfairly or unkindly or otherwise harmed if the money were spent to keep Pop comfortable. Was there anything nasty or selfish, if you stood in Pop's shoes, about spending the money this way?

They decided there wasn't. Pop and Mom had helped both kids when they were getting started in the world. By now, while neither child was exactly flush, both were certainly self-sufficient and perfectly willing to acknowledge that they'd had more than their share of their father's generosity. Spending the money on him, now that he had special needs, seemed like a good and decent thing to do.

As for Mr. Cantor's medical needs, John and Anne discussed possible future care scenarios with his physician and with a geriatric nurse-practitioner they knew. Both were extremely helpful—particularly their nurse friend, who was able to tell them what might happen through stories drawn from her own experience.

Not everyone, of course, is in a position to enjoy this kind of consultation. But some people don't recognize the resources they do have. Although busy health care professionals don't always initiate the necessary conversations with family members, they will often respond generously if someone in the family gets a discussion going. In addition, advice about nonmedical matters can sometimes be had from local Alzheimer's support groups and the local Agency on Aging. And there are plenty of written sources of information on specific practical issues such as keeping the person physically oriented and making the house safe, or that survey the entire range of problems. Some of these sources are listed at the back of this book.

Further Down the Road

During this process of putting together contingency plans, Anne's distrust of John decreased. She came to believe that he was really interested in doing the right thing, that he wouldn't weasel out of helping and wouldn't try to grab what he could for himself. They still had some disagreements, but Anne felt much safer than before, because she now believed there was no hidden agenda lurking beneath their arguments.

John, for his part, got a much better sense of Anne's needs. He started taking her fears about his sexism seriously. From the start, if you had asked him, "Should female relatives have to do more of the caring, just because they are female?" he would have answered, "Certainly not." But he did not yet see that, if he weren't careful, he might try to foist off extra chores on Anne—without realizing that he was falling into the very pattern he had consciously rejected. Seeing things from her point of view, however, soon made it clear to him how much Anne had at stake, and this gave him a more vivid idea of what shouldering his own fair share might mean.

The most important thing that happened was that, in spite of Mr. Cantor's unwillingness to talk about his future, his kids eventually got a better sense of what kind of care he would be comfortable with. This knowledge was going to be helpful when decisions had to be made down the road.

Mr. Cantor had told John emphatically that he didn't ever want to be hooked up to a machine that did his breathing for him. And everybody agreed they would never let this happen. But as their doctor explained to them, they were thinking about the matter too simply. Respirator-assisted breathing might be all wrong for Mr. Cantor if it merely made his dying a longer, more drawn-out business. It might be just *right* for him, though, if he were suddenly in a crisis situation where he needed a boost; in that case he might soon be able to breathe again on his own.

Actually, the doctor added, even this rule of thumb wasn't all that helpful. While you might want the respirator for an emergency tomorrow, after ten years with Alzheimer's, you might not want to bother any longer. The same is true for cardiopulmonary resuscitation (CPR). If Mr. Cantor's heart suddenly stopped beating tomorrow, CPR would be appropriate; in ten years, it definitely wouldn't be. But in between, there would be a considerable gray area. If John is supposed to make the call, to what should he look for guidance?

John and Anne, with their spouses and kids, resolved that they would look, not so much to rules or to procedures, but *to Pop:* the man they knew now and had always known, their father and grandfather, the man who was sometimes irritable but always decent and human. They thought they could find in the patterns of his earlier life, in his former likes and dislikes, in his personal style and moral convictions, the guidance they would need now that his care and his dignity were both in their keeping.

Is Advance Planning for Everyone?

Some people might feel that the Cantors' approach to the problem doesn't fit their own family very well. That may be because the family is already too burdened, or too spread out, or too dysfunctional to present any kind of united front against a dementing disease. But it may be because the Cantors' approach feels too formal, too idealized, too much like a business transaction. It may not feel enough like the way people in their own family relate to one another.

It's true that the Cantors' procedure is fairly formal. For Anne and John, it was useful to think of what they were doing as a special process, with special rules and procedures: Anne wrote down summaries of their discussions and got everyone, including her dad, to agree to what she had written. Such formality worked well for this family— as it might in your own—because the people within it didn't fully trust one another. The formality was a way of dealing with suspicion.

Anne was on her guard, concerned that old patterns in the relationship with her brother might reassert themselves, suspicious that her commitment to caring for her dad was greater than John's, fearful that she might be stuck with an unfair amount of work. The very fact that the decision making was given a special context made it easier for her to reconcile what she felt she owed her father, what she felt she owed other members of her family, and what she owed herself. John, too, found the approach comfortable; it reminded him a bit of the negotiations that sometimes went on at work, and because of that association he was more inclined to take the family conferences seriously.

But such an association, for many people, might be just the problem. For these people, caring for a loved one with dementia isn't just a job, and families aren't little corporations. "Negotiations" are what entrepreneurs do, not sisters and brothers, husbands and wives, parents and children. For people who feel this way, the special sense of solidarity and affection that can bind family members together and give them strength might seem undercut rather than strengthened by the "businesslike" atmosphere that worked for John and Anne.

Perhaps for some families, questions like "What shall we do when Dad is unable to bathe himself?" or "How do we decide when to take the car keys from Mom?" or "When should we stop life-sustaining medical treatment?" don't really arise. The traditions of these families are strong and clear enough so that these questions and others like them are already answered—or at least the *way* in which they'll be answered is clear.

For most families, however, we think the answers to these questions are not so clear. While their members are held together by ties of affection and obligation, there will still be conflicts, largely because these ties are so numerous and so important. It isn't simply parents or spouses that matter in our family lives. Our children matter, and our siblings matter, and we matter, and the decisions we make need to respect all those different connections.

Advance planning sessions within families shouldn't operate by the rules of the market, where you try to cut the best deal you can for yourself while the other guys look out for themselves. But if we are to succeed in gathering the family's strength, making the best possible decisions, and fairly apportioning the burdens, something like a deliberate and self-conscious process of sorting things out and coming to agreement is going to have to occur. There are good reasons to talk things over. As the Cantors discovered, where there's some kind of solidarity to build on, talking can not only restore trust, it can also help people who've known each other for years to come to a new understanding of who they are together.

3

A Semblance
of Normality

MARIE PYNE hates to be dependent on her husband Roy. *He* depends on *her*—always has—and that relationship isn't supposed to be turned upside-down. Besides, Marie really never has trusted him very much outside his own line of work. He was pretty good at operating earth-moving machinery, but that was about as far as it went. As for housekeeping or, years ago, taking care of the kids when they were sick, forget it.

He's got to take care of Marie now, though. She's been told that she has "dementia of the Alzheimer type," but she hasn't been able to take that fact in. Still, her dementia has progressed to the point where considerations of safety require Roy to keep a close eye on her. She's been burning herself regularly when she tries to cook dinner, and she finds that driving her car—even in daylight, even in her own neighborhood—is like entering a labyrinth.

Giving up the kitchen was a real hardship for Marie. She had been trying desperately to hang on, restricting her menu to simple meals, but the struggle was frustrating and painful. When Roy took away the microwave because she kept putting metal containers in it, she accused him of breaking it and hiding the pieces. She had always blamed him for being clumsy and stupid, so now, even though he knows she isn't responsible for what she says, her accusations hit home, hurting him the same way they always had. When he started unplugging the stove at night so she wouldn't burn herself while he was sleeping, he was careful to "fix" it in the morning with her watching—as if to prove to her that he wasn't clumsy and stupid after all.

For Marie, the idea of giving up driving was even more traumatic than curtailing her cooking, because of the loss of control and independence it represented. When Roy became convinced that she was starting to be a genuine hazard to herself and to other people, he tried to talk to her about it, but this made her frightened and defensive. It was no wonder, Roy thought. She was fighting to hang on to something crucial—her sense of herself as the person she'd always been. She wouldn't—couldn't—listen to Roy's pleading. For his part, he didn't like the idea of taking the car keys away from her by force. So for quite a while Roy simply made it his business to ride in the car with her any time she drove.

Roy was every bit as unwilling as Marie to see himself thrust into a caretaking role at his time of life. If anything, he tended to deny Marie's progressive loss of abilities longer than she did. The idea of his being "in charge" seemed as inappropriate and unlikely to him as it did to her.

The Pynes' career-oriented children, who live in distant cities, seem a little remote from their parents. There never was any one sharp break, no incident to which a person could point and say, "That's why their kids are so alienated." The fact remains, however, that Marie and Roy have been dealing with Marie's dementia on their own, except for Roy's niece Kathy, who stops by once or twice a week.

Marie's dementia is no longer merely a vague threat sending out ominous signals, but a daily reality, making everything about her life harder and more frightening than ever before. This is a time when Roy and Marie face difficult problems: for example, how to understand the shift in who is depending on whom, and how to balance risks to Marie—and to others—against the importance of helping her retain some degree of independence. The Pynes also face the challenge of defining what it means to live honestly together in the face of dementia. And as if all that weren't enough, Roy is taking on another new role: keeping faith with Marie's old self while he tries to understand and respond to her new reality.

Doing all this with grace will require a certain kind of thoughtful and imaginative caregiving, and Roy hasn't yet shown a great deal of enterprise in that direction. He could hardly be expected to, when he's got both hands full just struggling with the fact of his wife's illness. It's hard to summon up the sort of hope that spurs you to insight and creativity when you are facing a disease whose unavoidable conclusion is so profoundly depressing.

Despite his unpromising track record, however, Roy is slowly managing to come around. He is learning not merely to cope, but to do so with a kind of flair that surprises him as much as anyone. While still a reluctant cook and an indifferent housekeeper, he has come to an insight. He understands Marie's need to maintain what she can of the life she has always led, and, in small but important ways, he's being creative about how to help her do this.

Putting on fresh lipstick just before leaving the house was always part of Marie's daily routine—she didn't feel completely dressed without it. This had sometimes amused Roy, and sometimes (when it looked as if they would be late) slightly annoyed him. But most of the time he didn't think of it at all, until he started to notice that she couldn't get her lipstick on straight anymore.

One day she burst into tears as she struggled to do it. "My mouth is too little," she wailed. "I can't seem to aim at it today." Roy tried to help her, but the tube felt awkward in his hand and he had no idea how you put the stuff on, anyway. His incompetence only made things worse. Marie was too irritable to hold still for long. He felt he really *was* being clumsy and stupid, while she took his fumblings as fresh evidence of the fact that if she didn't do something herself, it wouldn't be done properly.

"I'm sorry, hon," Roy said after a few days of the lipstick wars. "I can't seem to get the hang of it. Does it really matter so much? You look fine without lipstick. Why don't you just stop wearing it?"

Marie couldn't stand this. Everything was being taken away from her, no matter how hard she tried just to be normal. Well, the world might be crumbling around her, but a lady never left the house without lipstick, and she wasn't about to start now. She could apply it herself if she had to. And she did. Badly.

Roy could have left the matter there, but the truth of it was that he was embarrassed by how she looked. He wasn't proud of this; he tried not to let it bother him; but she'd always been neat and tidy in her appearance, and now—! Besides, if he let her go out in public like that, people would start treating her differently, and that was the last thing she needed. So he'd have to come up with a second strategy. He'd just have to learn to use lipstick better.

He went into the bathroom, shut the door firmly, and practiced on his own lips until he got the hang of it. Brother, he thought, looking at himself in the mirror. Wouldn't the guys on the crew pay money to look at me now. All I need's a blond wig and falsies and I'm Marilyn Monroe. He grinned, washed off his mouth, and tried again. Having followed this up with a little extra experimentation on Marie, he can now apply lipstick for her with tolerable accuracy.

Something interesting happened as Roy learned a little cosmetology. Marie's daily routine became a shared ritual. She's grateful to him for helping her in this important way, and has begun to think he's not so clumsy after all. He's kind of handy, really. She supposes he could do some of the household chores she's tired of doing. And she likes having him put her lipstick on—it's kind of sexy, in a way.

Soon Roy got creative about other things as well. Marie had always been the "money person" in their house. Over the years, Roy brought home most of it, but it was always Marie who paid the bills, balanced the checkbook, and took care of the taxes. She struggled gamely on with these tasks too—longer than she should have, given the resulting confusions in their bank account. For a while, it looked as if the checkbook were going to have to go the way of the microwave. But now Roy has made it possible for her to feel that she is continuing to handle money, even though she is no longer up to it. He made a list of all the shops she was likely to patronize—her hairdresser, the grocer, the pharmacy. He made the rounds, explained the situation, and suggested a way Marie could continue to do business with them. Marie now pays for her purchases with checks that have been stamped "void." Her bills are actually sent to Roy every month, and he covers them out of his own account. He was concerned that the "void" stamp would give away the game, but Marie never seems to notice. It didn't occur to him that, although he was trying to be kind, these business people might start to treat Marie the way he'd feared they would if he let her go out of the house with her lipstick on crooked. That's just what the hairdresser did.

Sometimes Roy's bag of tricks is empty. Marie has occasional bouts of what would in a healthy person be considered bizarre nastiness. During a trip to the grocery store, for example, she suddenly began to shout at Roy. She yelled at him to go away and stop bothering her, telling the other customers that he was trying to steal her food. Roy was so distressed he couldn't even move, and simply stood there staring at her. Then she wrenched the cart away and started to slam it repeatedly into his shins. Mercifully, a neighbor who happened to be getting her groceries at the same time, was able to distract Marie. She soon forgot all about the frightening man who had tried to take her cart, and went home peaceably with her husband. This left Roy not only sore of shin, but extremely sore of heart. Marie's outburst angered and depressed him. It also scared him. His sense of who he was in relation to Marie had been a good part of what kept him going. His belief that he was doing a really good job of caring for her, much better than anyone could have anticipated, had been another source of strength. Now both of these beliefs were called into question. How could he continue to do a good job when she was nasty and abusive, and didn't even recognize him? Who *was* he in relation to this strange and ugly person? He hadn't realized her dementia was so advanced.

Changes

The ways in which Marie's and Roy's roles have shifted are painful, bewildering, and upsetting. The roles that make up our lives—particularly those we have lived with for years, and which absorb our time, energy, and creativity—become the pegs on which we hang our identities as the particular persons we are. When a dementing disease strikes, those basic roles change for both patient and caregiver, and identities can come unstuck.

Roy and Marie have to accept the fact that some changes are inevitable, and that all the kindness, empathy, and creativity in the world can't reverse the degeneration in Marie's brain. Some of her losses create problems the couple can't solve, problems that won't go away even if they can come up with the right strategies, get access to the right resources, enlist the support of friends and family. They are problems that Roy and Marie somehow must learn to live with.

For Roy, the main task became accepting what can't be changed with as little resentment as possible. This is never easy, and it has to be done day by day. As he struggled to live with what he couldn't fix, it struck Roy that maybe what he needed to do was to examine his ideas about what a human life is supposed to be like. Maybe he needed to change some of them.

This occurred to Roy when he visited a day care center shortly after Marie was diagnosed. Thinking that sometime in the future they might need such a program, he visited one that offered "stimulating and structured activities" to people with dementia while their family members enjoyed a little time off from caregiving. Through a window, he watched a group of women standing up and singing "You Are My Sunshine" while swaying back and forth to the music. The women were smiling and animated. In fact, to all appearances they were having a great time.

It was their very enjoyment that got to Roy. The idea that a person's life might come to *this,* that a person would be challenged and entertained by what looked like a kindergarten exercise, seemed to him disgusting and absurd. The idea that his own Marie was probably headed in that direction was bitter beyond words. At the same time, Roy also could see in these women a frightening image of himself in his own future, swaying back and forth and crooning half-remembered words to childish tunes.

However, as Roy watched one white-haired woman turn gracefully as she sang, something changed inside him. Suddenly, he simply couldn't see that woman, Marie, or himself as people who had completely lost their dignity. Perhaps, although it was sad, there was nothing especially awful about a dementing disease—not in the sense that it could really destroy a person's dignity. Dementia produces plenty of undesirable changes, Roy thought, but maybe not the loss of dignity. Maybe that's produced not so much by the disease as by having the wrong idea of what it is to be human. Maybe the lives of these smiling, singing, swaying women had frightened him because there was something the matter with his idea of what life was supposed to be. Many of us tend to blend our mental images of "dignified person" with our images of "productive, highly competent person," forgetting, perhaps, that none of us start out that way. We won't all end up competent, either. Maybe, Roy thought, the loss of competency isn't a cause for deep humiliation, but a part of the human story that may befall any of us. It's one way of experiencing the decline toward death. As such, it's a part of the poignancy and mystery of human life, not something outside humanity, not something completely foreign to us.

The change in Roy's outlook has done a lot to help him live day to day as Marie's disease worsens. Although he wasn't able to communicate his insight to Marie in words, the good effect it had on his own emotions did end up being communicated to her; the more calm and collected he could be, the less anxious and agitated she was. Roy had made a positive adjustment to change in his life.

While some changes have to be accepted through such adjustments in our images and ideals, others can be resisted, met more actively, influenced for better or worse. A major challenge in taking care of demented people is telling the difference between the two kinds of change. As we've observed before, family members can "cooperate" with dementia by treating an ill loved one in ways that speed up the loss of ability and self-concept. Or they can resist this process, finding new resources for extending abilities and improving attitudes. People's relationships, their very identities, are at stake in our responses to dementia. Making the distinction between what changes can be resisted or redirected, and what changes cannot, is a crucial part of the family caretaker's task.

She Might Get Hurt

Kathy came over to have a cup of coffee with her uncle Roy one day when Marie was at the day care center. She had an agenda. When was he going to take the car keys away from Aunt Marie?

"I'm terrified when I think of her on the road, even with you along. She'll kill you both one of these days." Kathy opened the drawer in the end table next to the couch, pulled out a coaster, and set her mug down on it. "It's over two years since she got lost driving home from my house that time. Don't you remember how frantic we were? I simply can*not* understand why you'd let her keep taking such risks."

"I know, I know. I worry about it all the time," Roy said. "But try to look at it from Marie's point of view. Think what it means to her."

"It means a car wreck waiting to happen," Kathy sniffed.

"It means she's normal," Roy contradicted, emphatically stirring a spoonful of sugar into his coffee. "It means she's an independent adult who can go places on her own and do things for herself like anybody else. If she can still get to the grocery store, she feels useful. She feels like she's still keeping house for me."

"Yes, but it's all playacting. She's *not* normal.

It's time to face facts, Uncle—she's not up to driving anymore."

"She's already lost so much, Kath," Roy pleaded. "She had to quit work, she doesn't see her friends much anymore, she doesn't get the pleasure out of cooking that she used to. If I take the car away from her, what's she got left? It's such a comfort to her that she can still drive. It makes her feel like things aren't so bad after all."

Kathy kicked off one shoe and drew her leg up under her, as if she were settling in for a long debate. "You're only thinking about Aunt Marie though, aren't you? What about all those other people who could lose their lives when she gets behind the wheel? It's sheer luck that she hasn't run over a little kid or had a head-on collision with somebody by now."

"Yeah, but everybody takes risks. They let fifteen-year-olds drive, even though most of 'em haven't got the sense God gave a canary. Taking chances doesn't have anything special to do with Marie being sick—*everybody* takes chances of one kind or another, every day, because that's the only way to get what you want. We live with risks all the time. The car companies have the know-how to make cars safer than they make 'em, but doing it would jack up the price, so we settle for 'safe enough.' And we know we could save lives if we lowered the speed limit, but we don't. We let people take chances."

"Within limits! We don't let babies play on the highway. At least most of us don't." Kathy reached for her mug and shot a withering glance at her uncle.

"Marie's not a baby," Roy said quietly. "She's a grown woman with a lot of dignity and she needs me to help her stay as strong and independent as she can. I'm trying to keep her from hurting anybody, and I think if I'm in the car I can do that. She's been so scared of losing her way that she doesn't mind having me ride with her so long as she can drive. If that changes—if it gets to where I can't count on her not to go off by herself—then I'll take her keys. But it'll hurt her."

The question of driving involved risk to other people. This was different from the question of cooking. Because Roy had done what he could to reduce the chances of fire in the kitchen, the only person Marie endangered there was herself. By not interfering with her when she continued to take that risk—apart from letting her know of his newly developed fondness for cold meals—Roy honored Marie's fullness as a person. Even more than the cooking itself, Marie valued her role as the one who fed her family. And there was another important part of her identity at stake here: she had never been the kind to be discouraged from doing something simply because there was discomfort or even danger involved.

So, although he really couldn't consult with

Marie about her "informed preference" concerning the danger versus the benefits of continuing to cook, Roy was guided by his memory of Marie's past, as well as his awareness of the continuing stake she had in maintaining her identity as the person who provided her family with meals.

As for her driving, although Marie continued to do it for quite a while after her dementia started to make itself felt behind the wheel, she limited herself more and more as time went on. Her biggest problem was always losing her way, rather than erratic or dangerous driving as such. With Roy in the car, the direction problem was solved, and avoiding driving in town, at night, or during bad weather lessened other dangers.

LIVING HONESTLY

It isn't enough to know when to continue risky activities and when to stop them. A loving caregiver will also be interested in cushioning the loss for the person who is ill with a dementing disease. Are there ways of helping that person hang on to the sense of importance and competence associated with activities that are no longer appropriate?

This was a question that interested Roy. It's why he made his special arrangement with the local merchants. While Marie couldn't be trusted to do the family books any longer, or to use a checkbook properly, she could be given the semblance of these responsibilities. Not only did Roy give her the checks stamped "void," he also got her a calculator with extra large keys and an especially bright display, to give Marie the sense that, despite her losses, she could still handle the finances. In fact, Roy took the whole thing over himself; the calculator was just a prop in the performance.

So Marie got to keep, longer than she otherwise would have, some things quite precious to her: a sense of usefulness and a feeling of continuity in a world that was changing with terrifying speed. Or at least she got to hang on to the *belief* that she had these things, and she was no longer in much of a position to distinguish what she believed from what was, in fact, the case. But without knowing it, Marie may have lost something else she had always prized: the kind of honesty that had consistently been a part of her relationship with Roy. In exchange for receiving the *impression* that she had kept her adult status, she may have lost the *reality* of being treated with the dignity and respect to which an adult is entitled.

There is, of course, another way of interpreting what has occurred. Her husband is creatively seeking a new vocabulary with which to express something that is true about Marie, but which cannot any longer be said in the old ways. Marie is still a person of substance and worth, as her history and present status attest. However, because of the handicaps that come along with her damaged brain, the typical ways of acknowledging her status simply don't work. Seen from this perspective, Roy's creative accommodations are ways to express a "deeper truth" about Marie, and, therefore, are not false or deceptive in any important sense.

What's the correct way to understand what is going on here? Is Roy trading off illusion for reality? If so, is it a good trade? Or is he using unusual means to express something that, fundamentally, is true? Sometimes Roy thinks he's been extremely clever about the whole thing, and that thought gives him some sorely needed affirmation of his ability to cope. But other times his stratagems make him nervous. How should he feel? Proud? Uncomfortable? Both? Neither?

Truth-telling has to be more the rule than the exception if we are to relate effectively to others. If deception were the prevailing practice, no one could trust anyone and much of our daily lives would be paralyzed. The amount of deception that does exist in daily life brings with it tremendous social costs.

But it seems equally true that a little judicious molding of the truth can sometimes have good effects. What Roy did with the neighborhood merchants has on the whole been extremely good for Marie, and there seems to have been only a little negative fallout. How could this possibly be faulted?

To get a perspective on the question, try to remember how you felt the last time you found out that someone had lied to you—even if the lie was "for your own good." It is likely your first thought wasn't, "Were the consequences of this lie good overall?" More probably, you felt hurt, offended, yanked around, manipulated by the deceiver—despite all the good intentions, and even despite good results.

This kind of response suggests that truth-telling has a dimension that reaches beyond immediate results, to the question of respect. Many people feel that to be the subject of deception—again, even in their own interests—is not to be treated with full respect. And when the person doing the deceiving is someone they have special reason to trust, they may feel that the covenant between them—the implicit promise to keep faith with each other—has been broken. Deceiving people is not wrong simply because it makes them feel bad: they feel bad because they were wronged. And anyway, it would be wrong even if they *didn't* feel bad.

Marie, most probably, won't feel bad. She is not going to see through any of Roy's deceptive strategies. But that doesn't mean he is honoring her dignity or treating her with the respect that is her due—especially considering that her dignity is already in a perilous condition.

For his part, Roy might reply that truth-telling is no longer the way to show respect for Marie, that being honest is made much more difficult because

of her dementia, and that we ought to cut him a lot
of slack as he tries hard to come up with ways of
making life easier for someone he loves. It's not
right to tell a lie so you can put somebody at an
unfair disadvantage, but that's very different from
deceiving a loved one in an effort to be kind.

If Roy said this he'd be right. But even lying out
of love can be an ethically dangerous strategy. For
one thing, there's something seductive about feeling that you are entitled to take liberties with the
truth. Lying to or deceiving others is a way of gain-
ing power over them, and that is surely an attractive idea to many of us much of the time. It can be
difficult to guard against this seduction, especially
if we feel forced to give in to it in one particular
area of our lives, as someone might who was caring for a demented spouse.

Further, many people would, if pressed to think
about it, feel some compunction about lying even
to children (as opposed to playing with them in
ways that blur fact and fantasy). Even assuming
that the children wouldn't penetrate the deception
and that some good end was in view, we might feel
we shouldn't lie. These scruples suggest that lying
raises moral problems even when the dupe is not a
fully rational and competent person.

Roy might make one last protest here. It's not as
if he deliberately set out to deceive Marie. She's got
these delusions that she's still able to make financial transactions. He's simply going along with her

because breaking down a demented person's delusions can be shattering.

Again, Roy is partly right. Breaking down a demented person's delusions can indeed be shattering, but going along with a delusion is rather different from helping to create one. When Roy rides with Marie in the car, he doesn't pretend he's not there so she can feel she's doing it on her own. When he gives her checks stamped "void," however, he's actively building on her delusional state.

Shading the truth—even outright lying—can achieve important goals for people in Roy's position. But it has its costs. It ought not to be seen as simply another routine strategy to be used, even with very kindly motives, when interacting with demented people. Insofar as possible, the presumption in favor of avoiding deceit ought to be seen as holding for demented as well as nondemented people.

CREATIVE COPING AND A SPECIAL KIND OF STRESS

We have seen Marie and Roy both making creative accommodations to their new situation, and finding some degree of success, of solace, even of renewed intimacy, in doing so. Routines have been ruptured, presenting Roy with a pointed invitation to think more seriously about his wife and what her life is like than he has done for a long time. As a partial consequence, he has been thinking somewhat less about himself.

This has been tremendously helpful to him as he has adjusted to his new life with Marie. The lipstick ritual is an excellent example of how creative coping has worked for them both. Roy has always said he'd do anything for Marie, but he never anticipated that "doing anything" might involve learning how to put on lipstick. However, thinking about Marie and her needs in a newly concentrated way brought him to it, and the result has been moments of closeness between them, moments they both cherish.

All these accomplishments—facing changes, managing risks, rethinking what it is to live honestly with each other, and creative coping—grew out of Marie and Roy's joint involvement in maintaining Marie's sense of self. What the two of them have to draw on for this task is the integrity of their relationship, their loyalty to each other, and Roy's loving imagination. Roy has become actively involved in maintaining his wife's sense of self, and therefore, we suggest, her actual personhood as well. Because people are, to some extent at least, formed and maintained by their interactions with others, they can also be eroded by the treatment they receive. If a person is thrust by others into the role of "senile old lady" it can become very difficult to resist this characterization and remain alive to other, equally valid characterizations. Marie may have dementia, but she is also a housewife, a mother, a neighbor, a friend. When she is in a fragile and confused state, she will require extra help from others to affirm these very important parts of herself that no one used to question.

There is, however, a special kind of stress lurking here, one that we will simply flag now, and explore in depth in later chapters. As Roy devotes more and more of his time, energy, and creativity to shoring up Marie's identity, what will happen to his own? Might it ever be the case that the demands and strains of caretaking become just so burdensome that he ought to refuse them?

Here, we aren't imagining conflicting duties to other people. Roy, fortunately, is pretty free of those. Rather, we are imagining conflicts *within Roy himself*. If a drastic change in her social context can help hold Marie together, in spite of her neurological disorder, might a drastic change in his social context pull Roy apart, in spite of his intact nervous system?

It's lucky in a way that Roy has not had the kinds of relationships and absorbing hobbies it would be painful to put on hold while Marie's care absorbs more and more of his time and attention. Nor is the task of caring for her so demanding that he literally has no time for himself. The Alzheimer day care program gives him some chance to recharge his own batteries. As we will see, however, not everyone is so well positioned, nor remains so all the way through the course of the disease.

4

From Home
to Nursing Home

ELAINE GIBBARD was diagnosed as having Alzheimer's disease five years ago. Her husband died the year before last, and about six months ago she moved into her son Alan's home. Alan lives in a small Cape Cod house with his wife Marjorie and their two daughters, Beth and Judy. Marjorie is an RN who works part time at the local hospital; Alan is an insurance adjuster; the kids are in high school.

Grandma Gibbard's arrival had a dramatic impact right from the start. For one thing, everybody lost their bedroom. The girls had to move in together, and as it made sense to put the two single beds into the master bedroom, Alan and Marjorie's double bed went into much smaller quarters. More pressure was put on the Gibbards' only—and already heavily trafficked—bathroom. Marjorie started to turn down extra shifts at work. Even the usual three a week became too much for her, and she could no longer be at the hospital when Alan was on the road.

To a large extent, these changes were anticipated and the family had done its best to prepare for them. Alan, Marjorie, Beth, and Judy had had a rather intense series of discussions just after Alan's father's death. At that point, Alan was pretty hesitant about asking Grandma to live with them, but there didn't seem to be any other choice. His sister and her husband had their hands full already with a chronically ill child and with layoffs at work, and it was clear that Grandma couldn't live on her own much longer. So Alan and Marjorie and the girls tried hard to anticipate just what would be involved in taking care of her, and to get their feelings squarely behind what they all saw as their duty.

But despite this careful preparation, having Grandma in their home wasn't at all what they had thought it would be. Whether it was the doubly disorienting blows of her husband's death and her change of residence, or whether her dementia had just progressed farther than anyone realized, Grandma brought with her some problems that caught the family off guard. Uninterrupted sleep has become a luxury at the Gibbards'. Grandma often gets up in the middle of the night and wanders through the house, getting panicky and crying uncontrollably until someone—almost always

Marjorie, unless she is at work—gets up and puts her back to bed. Dinner is no longer a welcome pause in the day's occupation, when people can relax, spend some time together, and catch up on each other's lives. Grandma needs too much help with eating. She can't get dressed by herself either, but that's not so bad; Marjorie lays out two outfits and, when Grandma has chosen one, helps her into her clothes. They used to have a dreadful time getting Grandma to brush her teeth, but now, instead of telling her to do it and thereby inviting refusal, Marjorie asks her to choose between the red and the blue toothbrush, and Grandma brushes more willingly. Harder to deal with is Grandma Gibbard's occasional incontinence. She can't always control her bladder. And what is worse is that sometimes she doesn't recognize her daughter-in-law, or even her son; the girls seem like strangers to her much of the time. This frightens her, and when she is frightened, she is often loud and aggressive.

Family life isn't totally grim, though. One day Alan came across his mother chatting happily with the lady in a hoopskirt who forms part of the wallpaper pattern in the upstairs hall. His first thought was to try to call her back to a better sense of her surroundings, but then it struck him that she seemed to be having a nice little talk and there was no reason to interrupt. And the other night, Grandma announced to the family that she was going out dancing. The reality, of course, is that Grandma isn't going dancing. Her dementia has progressed to the point where she can't even be left alone. And this in turn has had serious consequences for the Gibbards' social life.

Since she moved into her son's home, Grandma never sees any of her old friends, and it's not certain she would recognize them if they did make the trip to her new neighborhood. Alan and Marjorie never go out as a couple any more, and having people in for an evening has become difficult and rare. Even the family circle is sorely reduced after dinner. Beth and Judy vanish between dinner and bedtime, and are seldom to be found around the house during weekends or school breaks. Marjorie and Alan have only the vaguest impression of what their daughters' friends are like, since neither Beth nor Judy ever invites them over.

As the Disease Progresses

By this point in the Gibbards' lives, the answers to many questions—about sharing tasks, about balancing care for Grandma against care for other family members, about the kind of medical treatment that will be most appropriate down the road—have already been worked out. The Gibbards did a fair amount of advance planning and preparation, a fair amount of negotiating about who does what. However, even though thought and care were expended on these questions, the questions themselves have now shifted in both foreseen and unforeseen directions, so that the old answers are no longer workable. That means the questions have to be raised again and the responses reconsidered.

There is no possibility at this point of Grandma's being directly involved in such discussions, of course. But if, several years ago when she could still be included, Marjorie and Alan had anticipated the need to rethink old plans and to make new ones, they might have asked her how she'd want them to go about reconsidering things as time went on. Her answers then might make her family feel more comfortable with the decisions they must still make now.

Suppose, for example, there had been earlier discussions about where Grandma would want to live as the disease progressed, and she had chosen to live with Alan and his family. Suppose further that, during the discussion, someone had brought up the possibility that the family's caring resources could give out, and that a nursing home might at some point become necessary. If Mrs. Gibbard had explicitly acknowledged this possibility, then an eventual move of that kind might be easier on everybody.

The Gibbards' discussions took place too late for that. In any case, the family had focused more on the impact of her moving *into* the house, and less on the impact of her leaving it again. Clearly, the Gibbards have a lot more to talk about as the ongoing reality of Grandma's extended, day-to-day care becomes more and more a part of everyone's life.

But what they face is not merely a matter of coming up with new plans of action in response to steadily changing needs. It's also a matter of accepting something that can't be changed. The Gibbards, already stressed by the illness, now have to cope with two simultaneous trends, each of which is heartbreaking and which together are tragic. While Mrs. Gibbard's need for care continually expands, her ability to participate meaningfully in family life keeps contracting. She is moving toward a time when, like a newborn, virtually all of her needs will have to be met by others. Unlike a newborn, however, she won't possess the vital sense of future promise, of new abilities flowering daily, that almost all babies have. And there is nothing her family can do about this.

The Gibbards, then, are faced with a huge challenge. How can they protect what they value about their life with Grandma when she is passing beyond the point of being able to recognize and interact with them? How can they come to terms with what is happening to this person they love? And how can they make the hardest decision they've ever faced as a family—entrusting

Grandma to a nursing home? In this chapter, we will focus on all these problems.

"WEAR AND TEAR" VS. "ADAPTATION"

"What I'm worried about," remarked Marjorie to Alan late one afternoon as Grandma dozed in front of the TV, "is that if we keep this up much longer we're going to wear ourselves right out. Keeping your mom from wandering off is getting to be a full-time job and we're all heading toward exhaustion. And look at how tense things are between us and the kids. I've been having one cold after another all winter, which is nothing but stress. You've been getting headaches. And Judy flunked math last term. At some point, the wear and tear on the family is going to be so enormous that we won't be able to keep Grandma at home anymore, and what'll we do then?"

Alan took two beers out of the refrigerator and reached for the bottle opener. "What'll we do?" he repeated. "We'll adapt. We'll grow. We'll learn how to cope with the challenges as they get more challenging." He poured beer into a glass and watched it foam up. "See, I think you've got the wrong idea about what people can stand. It's not like they only have X amount of care and compassion in them, and if somebody drains it all out before they fill it back up again, they're empty.

That's more like a gas tank than a person. Or like this beer glass. What're you, a beer glass?"

Marjorie took the glass and drank from it. "Better that than a gas tank, I guess. Remind me again why I'm not a beer glass?"

"Because you can expand your caring capacity. You can cultivate your resources until you've got more than you ever thought you could have. I've seen you do it. You're wonderful, Marge. You started out very loving, but dammit if you haven't grown about six sizes this last year. You aren't going to wear out or drain out. You'll just adapt."

"Yeah, well, maybe I do adapt. But I've been doing more than my share and I'm tired. How about you getting off your duff and growing a couple more sizes too? You can start by getting Grandma back to bed tonight."

Obviously, Marjorie didn't share Alan's rosy view, but as they kept talking, she came to think that maybe they both were right. Maybe she and Alan could keep up the home-based caregiving for the period of time when it was most important to Alan's mom. Maybe for just that long the family could keep adapting enough to shoulder the task. And maybe after a while, when that task became so heavy it really would wear them all out, when Grandma's care started to destroy other important parts of their lives, maybe then it would seem natural and appropriate to let the brunt of the care pass on to professionals. She'd feel awfully guilty about it, though.

Anyway, as Alan pointed out, they all *had* adapted. They had all been changed by the caregiving they'd been doing. Changes in routine had themselves become routine. What at first seemed like extraordinary problems become decidedly ordinary. But the idea wasn't just that people can get used to anything. Rather, Alan was arguing that providing care for his mom had transformed the caregivers. In his opinion, the experience of giving basic and intense care itself deepens and widens what the caregiver can do, and even who the caregiver is.

What happened, of course, is that the Gibbards both adapted *and* experienced wear and tear. The many tasks of caregiving became progressively less distressing but also more difficult. After a time, like other loving, well-motivated, and conscientious caregivers, they did simply become exhausted. Their own health got worse and their ability to honor other commitments was strained. Now the problem is figuring out how they can reduce wear and tear while increasing their ability to adapt, so that they can at least survive sharing their home with Grandma. Because they're still concerned about responding well to her great need, this is a moral question as well as a practical one.

WHERE THE RESOURCES CAN BE FOUND

One essential part of the Gibbards' strategy must be to get help from their community. They need to learn about sources of support, both practical and psychological. There may be ways to get temporary help that would allow Alan and Marjorie to get out together now and then. Perhaps there are affordable senior day care facilities that Mrs. Gibbard would like and that would make it easier for the girls to have their friends over. They can get information about these sources of help by phoning their local Agency on Aging or the Alzheimer's Association.

There may also be resources the family can tap into at home. Mrs. Gibbard's new environment may become less disorienting as she becomes more familiar with it, or even as she loses the ability to note the difference between the familiar and the strange. If letting a little time pass doesn't ease her disorientation, there may be changes and adjustments that her family can make in the home. Lights can be left on in hallways at night. The CD player can still play grunge rock bands, but also Grandma's old favorite—Mario Lanza singing songs from *The Student Prince*. And Mrs. Gibbard can be included in the daily chores that are familiar to her: whoever is putting dinner together or washing up afterward can take her into the kitchen, too.

Finally, there are resources in Alan, Marjorie, Beth, and Judy themselves, ways of thinking and feeling that may help to nurture their own caregiving inclinations and abilities. New ways of thinking about a situation are resources that can make it easier to respond (as Roy found out in the last chapter) without feeling defeated or devastated. And other inner resources can make it possible to stay better connected—both to the person who so often doesn't act or look like her old self anymore, and to one's own self, as well.

STAYING CONNECTED

Marjorie first figured out how to do what she calls staying connected to herself one day twenty years ago, shortly after she saw that she would have to give up the baby she was carrying for adoption. She hadn't meant to get pregnant—she was still in school, struggling to keep up her grades, with no prospects for her life unless she got her degree. Her boyfriend wanted to help, but he was as much of a kid as she and no better equipped for fatherhood than her sixteen-year-old brother. Her parents wouldn't take her in; she had nowhere else to turn. But how could she leave her own wonderful baby with strangers? It would tear her apart.

It was while she was numbly walking to class

one day in the middle of all this that she realized she could relate to herself as a deeply concerned, benevolent friend—a friend who loved her very much. From that viewpoint, she could feel enormous compassion for this young woman plodding along the sidewalk, wishing her well as she journeyed one year, five years, ten years down the road. It didn't take away the numbness in her legs or the pain in her heart, but it did seem to put it all into a richer context, one that made it easier for her to get unstuck, to start moving again with some sense that she wasn't completely alone, and that her life was very much worth living.

She has never gotten over the pain of having to give her baby up for adoption, but ever since, this memory of good friendship has been useful to Marjorie when she goes through difficult times. However hard her life may be, she always retains the sense that she is connected and not alone. And this sense, in its turn, helps her get through her troubles with more grace and less damage, less wear and tear, than she otherwise might experience.

When Marjorie was walking to class that day, it seemed to her that she had found a way of looking at her life that was both intimate and deeply engaged. She knew just what was going on, and she wasn't distorting how she felt about it. These weren't feelings of heroic self-denial, nor feelings that her problems were trivial compared to what others were going through, nor feelings of loyalty to the eternal verities, nor anything of that sort. She was buoyed up by her friendship for herself, but in a way that wasn't totally self-absorbed or dominated by the problem she faced at that moment in time. Rather, she allowed her loving concern for her own life and what was happening within it to spill over her tragedy and fit it into a broader vision.

What Marjorie experienced then was not simply a refined sort of egotism. She also started to see those around her in a more connected way, and hence, more sympathetically. She now knows that releasing whatever inner resources she has available to help her is in large part a matter of embracing the people in her life—including her mother-in-law—richly and deeply. Alan and the children have long been aware of this strategy for connecting to herself like a friend when times are hard. Can they, like Marjorie, achieve a perspective from which to "connect" to their sometimes nasty and always upsetting Grandma?

All the Gibbards have tried to cultivate this kind of connection these past several months. Mrs. Gibbard's presence in their home has been disruptive, distressing, difficult, and damaging. Despite their best efforts, they are all rather less in touch with one another than they were at this time a year ago, and everyone is feeling a sort of pervasive sadness. But they do realize that they are a part of something deeply important: the closing chapter in the life of someone they all love. Somehow, business as usual is just not fitting at such a time. Right now, life for the Gibbards is hard and sad—and at the same time, an invitation to love.

Because they've tried hard to reconnect themselves to their situation, Beth and Judy don't find it as shameful and socially upsetting as they did at first. Judy started thinking about how she'd react if all this were happening to a close friend, and on the strength of her reaction she found the courage to invite a few of her more thoughtful and sensitive friends home. She hasn't regretted it, even though one of her friends found it too uncomfortable an experience to want to repeat. At first that made Judy mad, but then she had to laugh at herself, since feeling "uncomfortable" was precisely why she herself had been staying away from home so much. As a result of her experiment, Judy's been able to cut her friend some slack—and cut herself some, too.

The effort to stay connected also helps everyone maintain a more vivid sense of Mrs. Gibbard than they otherwise might have. Rather than simply focusing on the old woman here and now—a woman who is being obstreperous, or a lot of trouble, or who doesn't seem to know these people who are all breaking their backs to take care of her, they keep in mind that Grandma brought with her into the present moment a full history, one in which all their own lives are deeply engaged. The family has tried to nourish this way of thinking by ransacking old albums and "keepsake" boxes for pictures, cards, and other mementos of Grandma's life, and the life they have shared together. Old photos have been dusted off and put in new frames around the house.

Staying connected to Grandma and to each other has made a difference in the family's experience of caring for her, and for one another as well. It isn't magic, of course; their situation remains difficult, distressing, and even damaging. But the grace that is growing allows them to feel the importance of what they're doing. It may extend their career as her primary caregivers. And it may also ease their own transition to a different kind of caretaking role, when and if Mrs. Gibbard leaves to take up residence in a nursing home.

THE NURSING HOME

Many of us dislike the thought of nursing homes, not only because of the not-so-distant scandals that have been associated with them, but also because they make us feel we've failed. The popular image of these homes has a lot to do with their history, which traces back to the poorhouses of the nineteenth century. It was a disgrace to have to go to the poorhouse—a sign of thriftlessness and lack of moral fiber. Shame attached to families who were so improvident as to be forced to resort to such places for care. Yet poorhouses, grim and punitive though they were, increasingly became a dumping ground for the old and infirm.

At the beginning of the twentieth century, state mental hospitals seemed like a more humane alternative, at least for the care of the demented elderly. At the same time, medical hospitals came to specialize in short-term, acute care. Nursing homes, some sponsored by churches and some intended to turn a profit, began to provide long-term care—increasingly, the care of the old. At mid-century, when the deinstitutionalization movement prompted state mental hospitals to discharge many of their aged residents to communities that, as it turned out, could not care for them, nursing homes became even more specialized. They became places where elderly people suffering from dementing diseases could go.

In the 1950s and 1960s, just at the time when mental hospitals were releasing their elderly patients, scandal after scandal gave nursing homes an even worse name. There were widespread reports of substandard care and outright physical abuse. There were shady financial practices, ranging from kickbacks and fraud to theft of residents' assets. Strict governmental oversight in the last fifteen years has begun to correct these evils, but the truth is that many nursing homes are still rather bleak and depressing places. Residents sometimes injure

other residents or take their things; daily life can
be extremely tedious and boring in the absence of
structured activities; the surroundings can be grim
and utilitarian; staff can be unresponsive or disrespectful of the person who is ill; and in even the
best of homes there is no getting away from the
clamor, the lack of privacy, the totality of the institution. The stigma of the poorhouse remains attached to nursing homes, and families still tend to
blame themselves for having to "abandon" a loved
one to them.

As it stands now, only 5 percent of the elderly
spend any length of time in nursing homes, although that number will increase as the baby
boomers grow old. Moreover, family abandonment of the elderly is relatively rare in the United
States, where heavy care, often past the point of
burnout, is the _norm_ for family relationships.
Most families will not consent to nursing home
placement until their own caregiving capacities are
exhausted, even though this is hard on both the
frail elderly person and her or his family. The
avoidance of institutional care is understandable.
Nursing homes still summon up images of neglect,
abandonment, and poverty, even though there
have been significant attempts at reform.

The Gibbards found the idea of a nursing home
so distasteful that they initially ruled it out altogether. They'd been having a hard time sorting
through negative stereotypes and false pride when-

ever the subject came up. Finally, though, they reconsidered. They came to realize that at some
point they might not be able to meet all of Mrs.
Gibbard's needs, and they toured a facility that
looked as if it could meet them. But they weren't
ready to decide anything yet.

When the Time Comes

Then one Saturday night Alan came home to find
the family in an uproar. That afternoon when
Beth, who had been the only one home with Mrs.
Gibbard, was in the shower getting ready for an
evening out, the old lady had wandered outside
and disappeared. She had now been missing for
more than five hours, and everyone was frantic.
Marjorie had called the police and the two hospitals in town, but no one had seen anyone answer-
ing to Mrs. Gibbard's description.

The police eventually brought her home. Despite the latches Alan installed high up on all the
doors leading outside, which everyone tried hard
to remember to secure, the same thing happened in
the middle of the night two weeks later. This time
it was Alan who found her—in her nightgown in
the snow, two miles from the house. "I was trying
to go home," she sobbed. "I can't find Daddy."

After he and Marjorie warmed her and got her
to bed, it was Alan's turn to cry. "I'm doing a
lousy job of taking care of her, Marge. She's miser-

able and homesick and I don't know what to do about it. And look at you—you're worn out. What she needs is somebody with her all the time, day and night. And we haven't got the money for that, because I don't have a good enough job. Goddammit, I feel like I'm letting everybody down!"

Marjorie knew he wasn't letting anybody down and tried to tell him so. She didn't feel as angry as he, but she could match him guilt for guilt. She felt she was doing everything wrong, that she was failing, that this lovely woman who had always been so good to her and who was now so needy and vulnerable deserved far better than she was getting. And she also knew that she and Alan were in treacherous, unspoken agreement that the time had come to find a nursing home.

Treachery was the operative emotion here. They felt they were betraying Mrs. Gibbard. Surely, they thought, we could be working at it a *little* harder than we are. Surely we aren't giving 100 percent. Surely we could buy her just a little more time with us if we were more patient and less lazy. These emotions were strongest in Alan, of course, since it was his mother, and because of that, Marjorie didn't feel she could take the initiative. She could only look on, guilty, as Alan struggled with his feelings.

It was Judy who broke the impasse. She and Alan were sharing a late night snack at the kitchen table, waiting for Marjorie to come home from work. "You think Grandma's going to have to go to a home, don't you?"

"She's not going to a home. I promised her we'd never do that, and we're not going to."

"Yeah, but it's not that simple, is it? So you're wondering how you're going to live with your-self."

Alan didn't say anything. Judy pushed her plate aside and propped her elbows on the table. "I've been thinking about it, Daddy. Listen. You know how when there's a divorce, little kids are afraid that if their parents can stop loving each other, they could stop loving *them?* It doesn't work like that, but that's what little kids think. They get mixed up about what counts as a divorce and what doesn't." She smiled at him sadly, her face glowing in the lamplight. "If you put Grandma in a nursing home, you aren't divorcing her. It's a big change in the family, but it's not a divorce. You don't stop loving her. It doesn't work like that. It's pretty easy to get mixed up about it, though."

That moment was an important one for Alan. It didn't put an end to his guilt or allay his anger, but it unstuck him so that he and Marjorie could get serious about finding a nursing home that would meet his mother's needs. They checked out the six that were close enough for frequent visits, thinking these would be crucial for everyone's peace of mind. What they didn't know then, but were soon to discover, is that frequent visits were also important for building rapport with the nursing home staff. Residents who had family to communicate, translate, and advocate for them generally got better and more individualized care than those who didn't. The reason is that families serve as historians of a kind. They can tell the staff who this person had been: "She's too quiet. That's not like her. Maybe she's depressed, or not feeling good, or something's bothering her." By their presence, families can also set the staff an example of loving and respectful care.

For these reasons, the home had to be close by. But it also had to feel okay. Marjorie and Alan crossed three off the list right away because they felt unfriendly or unkempt or just—funny. Of the other three, St. Anne's had a Dementia Special Care Unit, designed to maintain residents' functioning as long as possible, and then, when the disease was advanced, to promote people's comfort rather than treat them with inappropriate, aggressive medicine. The Gibbards thought this facility would be better for Mrs. Gibbard than the others, so they put her on the waiting list.

They dreaded telling her, and when they did, it was as bad as they feared. First she cried, and then she yelled, and then she insisted that they get out of her house. By the next day, though, she had forgotten, so they let it alone temporarily. They hired an elder lawyer to help them do the paperwork and sort out the financial side of things. He was expensive but worth it, because he knew what needed doing and they didn't. When it was all done, they waited.

When the call came, they packed up Mrs. Gibbard's things and once again tried to explain to her where they were going. She couldn't seem to understand until Beth said, playfully, that they were taking her to a college where she'd learn to improve her memory. Alan shot her a very black look, but Grandma was interested. "College?" she beamed. "You know, I always wanted to go to college. Let's get in the car!" Rattled, but amused all the same, Marjorie and Alan helped her in and drove her to St. Anne's.

Leaving her there was dreadful. Alan was wracked by guilt and Marjorie felt she could never look her mother-in-law in the face again. There were so many old and ill people about, and some of them were making noises. Grandma's roommate seemed nice enough, but she followed Marjorie around wherever she went, and Grandma looked little and bewildered. But she told her roommate proudly, "I'm in college now." And while Alan felt he shouldn't let her keep thinking that, he also needed desperately to make things easier for her, and couldn't bring himself to correct her belief.

In the Nursing Home

The Gibbards visited Grandma regularly—twice a week for a while. Although Alan got off to a bad start with the regular staff by being critical and demanding, Marjorie could see that Grandma was losing out because of this, and persuaded him to save his criticisms for things that really mattered. "The aides are only human," she urged. "Like anybody else, they do their work much better if they're admired and appreciated. Connect with them—you know yourself it's not easy looking after old people." They brought pictures of a younger Grandma to give the nursing home workers some sense of the whole of her life. They tried hard to supplement the direct knowledge the staff had of her now with their own knowledge of her past.

They learned it was also good to visit on the weekends, when the auxiliary staff was on duty. One Saturday when Alan arrived he found his mother wearing a diaper, due to a weekender's mistake. "Mom!" he exclaimed. "You don't need a diaper. Why didn't you tell the aide?"

"Oh, I thought they were trying something new."

For a time, Mrs. Gibbard actually seemed to do a little better than she had at home—partly because of the special programs in the dementia unit and partly, perhaps, because she was no longer in the sole care of exhausted and burned-out relatives. But after a year or so the days on which she was withdrawn, critical, and angry began to outnumber the "good" days, and visiting her came to be a real chore.

Marjorie and Alan were faithful about it, though. They were now visiting only once a week, but it *was* once a week, and Judy and Beth came once or twice a month. Conversations with Grandma were—well, weird—because she would say disconnected and cryptic things and you never knew who you were to her. Sometimes Beth was Mrs. Gibbard's daughter, sometimes her sister, sometimes her mom. And it was the same for Marjorie. It was easier if two or more of the family came together, because then they could at least talk to each other. It was also easier to visit together in Mrs. Gibbard's room than in the residents' lounge, because when she was in the lounge she felt the need to get up and look after the other visitors, bringing them magazines or the potted plants on the tables, or pulling up chairs for people to sit on.

Over time, the family got to know the other residents and some of their relatives, although not everyone had family to come and visit. Marjorie and Alan made a point of smiling and speaking to everyone, even though this sometimes invited more attention from a resident than they had bargained for. And almost every week Mrs. Rizzuto would come into Mrs. Gibbard's room when they were there and lie down on the roommate's bed. She couldn't speak much English, but Marjorie and Alan would nod and smile to her, and when the visit was over she would go back to her room. It seemed she needed visitors too.

As disconcerting, distressing, and upsetting as their visits could be, Alan and Marjorie continued to come. They could see it made a difference to the staff, not only because it was a way of keeping an eye on Mrs. Gibbard's care, but because faithful visiting demonstrated that they had a certain amount of "sweat equity" invested in Mrs. Gibbard's welfare. It gave them standing with the nursing home staff. They were listened to better than family members who came only a few times a year.

The Gibbards didn't visit simply as a means of maintaining good relations with Grandma's caregivers, however. Nor was it guilt alone that compelled them to come. These motives played their part, to be sure, but had they been magically removed, Marjorie and Alan, Beth and Judy would still have made their way to St. Anne's on a regular basis. It was a part of their covenant with Grandma. It was a way of keeping connected to her.

5

The Final Stages

RANDOLPH WOLTER, born in 1911, lost his father to the influenza epidemic that swept the country soon after Armistice Day. He weathered the Depression, which broke just as he was trying to get into the job market, and when war was declared after Pearl Harbor, he threw over his job at the garage and joined the Navy. He spent his war as a Seabee—a construction engineer—hopping from atoll to atoll in the Pacific Theater. His ship was nearly torpedoed once, he had a couple of minor construction accidents, and he came down with a nasty bout of malaria. None of that was particularly traumatic, but when enemy fire killed one of his buddies, a guy he'd grown particularly close to and who died in his arms, he couldn't seem to get over it. He talked of it often in later years—of how it frightened and enraged him.

After the war he went back to his hometown,

where he kept on working in construction. It was tough work, and though he never again was knocked out by a falling pylon, there were a lot of inconveniently timed layoffs as the fortunes of the economy ebbed and flowed over the years. Given the choice between construction accidents on the one hand and being out of work on the other, he figured he'd just as soon take his chances with falling pylons. He fell in love, married, and started a family. He was a volunteer firefighter, owned his own home, and did a fair amount of fly fishing. He had, as he used to put it, "a pretty good time, taken all in all."

The good times seem very long ago now. Mr. Wolter, for many years a widower, has been suffering from a multi-infarct dementia (caused by a series of little strokes) for over ten years, and it's been a long time since he's been able to interact with his family at all. His three children still live nearby, and if you asked them, they'd say they were a pretty close family.

Mr. Wolter's children managed to keep him out of the nursing home for quite a long while. Their mom's mother spent some time in a home just before her death, and though they were only kids at the time, they remembered the smell of stale urine and the tight-lipped nurses, and it left them with a bad attitude toward such places. That was why all three of them tried to take turns with their father's care. When Mr. Wolter was no longer able to live on his own, his house was sold and he moved in with his eldest son Paul and Paul's wife Rebecca. He lived with them for almost two years and then moved on to live with Amy, his favorite child, for better than five years. Then he lived briefly with Randy. Everybody helped as best they could. During the long and taxing time he lived with Amy, Paul or Randy would sometimes come over and spend a few days with him while she took a little break. This pattern continued for the two months he lived with Randy.

Mr. Wolter's doctors had advised against shuffling him around too often, stressing that he would do best in a stable, highly structured environment, and that changes in residence—or even changes in who was taking special responsibility for his care—could quicken the disorienting, disabling impact of his illness. So Mr. Wolter stayed about as long as possible at every stop, living with each child until the wear and tear got to be too much. Whether because of being shuffled around, or simply because of his dementia, things were particularly difficult during his years with Amy. He kept wandering away from home, and then toward the end of his stay, he became increasingly unpleasant and violent. That's when Randy agreed to take him. But it didn't work out. Shortly after he arrived at Randy's house, Mr. Wolter knocked him over, hitting him so hard that Randy broke a table as he fell. At that point, there was no help for it.

Randy took him to the emergency room for a psychiatric evaluation, after which he was pronounced a danger to himself and others and admitted to a psychiatric hospital.

After thirty days, although Mr. Wolter was still violent, the hospital staff told Randy they were going to release him. Appalled, Randy called his family doctor, who informed him that it was illegal in that state to discharge a psychiatric patient without a discharge plan—a plan for the patient's continued care. So Randy called the hospital's executive director, explained the situation, and requested a plan. The hospital then discharged Mr. Wolter to one of the few nursing homes in the area willing to take combative patients. Cedarcrest wasn't an ideal home by any means, but it was all there was. That was three years ago.

Mr. Wolter is by now extremely ill. It's been a long time since anyone has heard him say anything that could count as a clearly recognizable word, let alone put a sentence together. He can stand, but not move very much. He's been having increasing problems with swallowing his food, and he drools a good deal. It's been more than two years since he had any control of his bladder or bowels. Because his children don't think much of Cedarcrest, they've haunted the place in an effort to make sure their dad's care is okay. Randy and Paul have been spending time with him several days a week. Amy is there at least every other day. They are sad to see him so ill.

The demanding but relatively smooth routine into which matters had fallen was abruptly shattered one morning when a staff member called Amy. Mr. Wolter had developed a serious urinary tract infection and was comatose. He had been taken by ambulance to a nearby hospital—the one where Amy was born—and was on a respirator in the intensive care unit (ICU), with every effort being made to get his infection under control. Amy phoned her brothers from the hospital, breaking the bad news and assuring them that the ICU team was doing everything they could to keep their dad going. Paul and Randy, however, seemed less than enthusiastic about this course of action. Both brothers thought that what Dad would have liked best was simply to die at home. Amy, caught off guard by her brothers' attitude, opposed them bitterly. She said they were just tired of going to see Dad and wanted him to die, not for his own sake, but for theirs. She set the receiver in its cradle with a little more force than was strictly necessary and marched off to the ICU.

There, a few weeks later, he still remains. He's no longer connected to a respirator, but he has several other tubes sticking out of him. Amy is standing at his bedside, holding his hand, weeping quietly. Behind her, Paul and Randy are talking in low tones with the attending physician. Mr.

Wolter has stopped eating, and the question now is whether a feeding tube should be surgically inserted in his abdomen. The doctor has already explained that, along with more and more of his colleagues, he's reluctant to place a tube when the patient is severely demented, because it's somewhat uncomfortable and prolongs the process of dying. Amy knows her brothers wouldn't be in favor of the surgery even if the doctor recommended it and that, without it, their father won't live much longer. Amy knows too that pretty soon they'll ask her what she thinks. Standing there next to her unresponsive father, she doesn't know what she should say.

We discuss two themes in this chapter. The first is familiar: what is the role of the family in maintaining the selfhood of the demented person? Although this is a question we've never been far away from in this book, it seems particularly difficult to answer now that this final stage has been reached. This deep into the course of dementing disease, families will feel they have little to work with. It isn't merely speech and mobility that have gone; people as ill as Mr. Wolter don't seem to be themselves anymore. In fact, they don't seem to have an identity at all. Even now, however, the family has important maintenance work to do. And this work of maintaining the demented person's selfhood is crucially connected to our second theme: making decisions about health care at the end of life.

Maintaining Selfhood for the Deeply Demented

Families are a source of selfhood, consisting of perhaps the most fundamental set of relationships in the context of which people's identities are formed. Many of our core values, our strategies for coping with the world, and our basic personality styles come from our family upbringing. Many of us also find in our families the ongoing connections that reinforce and renew these parts of our identities—and even provide us with a certain degree of safety as we challenge and experiment with who we want to be.

Families start this work of forming our identities when we are babies. When we are grown, through the many subtle and not-so-subtle ways in which our intimates respond to us, they show us who they think we are: the constant mirroring we get from those with whom we interact most closely is an important mechanism by which we maintain our sense of ourselves. Families can also be a special home for human selves at the far end of life— the place where the person continues to exist even after his own body has ceased to be a home to him, even after he is no longer aware of the world around him, of those who love him, and of himself at the center of it all.

By telling stories in this book we have tried to show how people's lives can be seen as complicated, interconnecting lines of plot and character, arranged in patterns we can make sense of, and that others can understand. Understanding a loved one's life story allows us to make decisions about his health care in accordance with what the loved one would have wanted, *because* he would have wanted it; this process is an important way of keeping the patient connected to his own story. Even when the actual decision cannot or should not be solely the patient's—other people count too, after all—families can make decisions that take the ill person's character seriously. By maintaining a vivid sense of their relative's personhood in the process of making decisions that affect them all, the family can keep their relative "alive" as a member of their own intimate community, even after this person has passed beyond all knowledge of their love.

One source of the family's authority to make medical decisions for a loved one is that they have a stake in what's decided. But there is another source of decision making authority: the family's ability to reveal who their loved one has been and still is when his own actions are no longer self-revealing.

E. M. Forster's novel *Howards End* concerns what happens when the dying Mrs. Wilcox bequeaths her beloved home, Howards End, to Margaret Schlegel, an acquaintance to whom she has become very attached. The Wilcox family, appalled at the thought of an outsider taking possession of the family property, suppresses Mrs. Wilcox's will. In due course, Margaret ends up owning Howards End anyway, because she becomes the second Mrs. Wilcox. But that doesn't mean that everything has come out as it should. The wrong has not been righted, because the first Mrs. Wilcox didn't simply want Margaret to *have* Howards End—she wanted to *give* it to her as her gift, as an expression of her affection. Had the family honored her will, they would, in a sense, have acted in a way that showed something important about Mrs. Wilcox.

Not every family, of course, is equally well equipped to act in a way that expresses something significant about their loved one's personality. Families consist of individuals with separate, as well as shared, histories and hopes. While the connections among family members may be strong, they also might, as we have seen, contain very different agendas, deeply rooted suspicions, old grievances. And even when such considerations do not figure prominently in the equation, family members will grieve and love in their own different ways. What are sometimes called "moral emotions"—guilt for one, compassion for another— will be much in evidence as family members gather at the bedside. If individual needs and feelings aren't recognized and addressed, the final stages of the loved one's dying may be harmful to everyone involved.

Further, family members are not only in relationships with one another and with their demented and dying loved one—they are also in a relationship with the health care system. The tie between families and the institution of medicine is of profound importance, for it involves, at the moment of death, the family's understanding of the meaning of this event and the place of medicine in it. If all has gone well, the family will have discussed death with the patient long ago. They will have had family conferences and perhaps will have the patient's advance directive to guide them. But they must also revisit those questions in the light of their intervening experience.

Is it a legitimate goal of medicine to extend Mr. Wolter's life as long as possible? If his children really loved him, wouldn't they insist on the medical team's doing everything they could for him? What is the connection between withholding medical treatment and abandonment? What are the natural limits of human life, and how far ought we or dare we to press them? As we reflect on these general questions, we'll discuss some ideas that families can use to build their own particular paths through this difficult terrain.

FAMILY DECISION MAKING AT THE END OF LIFE

Mr. Wolter's children face decisions that are even tougher than people might think. For one thing, *everybody* in the family is on to something important in their thinking. Paul and Randy find it very hard to imagine what kind of good anyone could get out of a life like the one their dad has. He is, to put it bluntly, incapable of doing, thinking, or even feeling almost anything. Besides, his death can't be long delayed. Even if there is some value attached to living the way he is, Mr. Wolter won't be losing much if this episode of illness rather than some later one takes him away. And when you consider just what surviving this episode might cost him in terms of the pain and discomfort that accompany even minor surgery—pain he can't make sense of and doesn't understand—the meager good that such a life might be to him is surely outweighed by the rigors of being scanned, prodded, probed, injected, cut, and otherwise disturbed in order to prolong it.

These are all weighty considerations. At the same time, Amy is quite right to feel that neither brother's motivation here is completely unselfish. Dad has been difficult to take care of, and it isn't easy to regard this as rewarding work when he's so completely unable to acknowledge what they're doing. It isn't clear to either brother that the care they've been giving has really benefited him in any meaningful sense over the past few years. To one extent or another, they both feel their father has already died. "He passed away years ago," Paul says sorrowfully, "and left a disgusting stranger in his place."

If their care is costing them so much and offering him so little, what could be wrong in deciding that it's time to let Mr. Wolter go? Amy means very well, her brothers allow, but they see her as having invested so much in her father's care that she's not clear about the boundaries here. Randy put it this way: "Amy thinks that if we don't keep Dad alive as long as we can, we're telling her she's a failure, and that all her hard work went for nothing."

Randy isn't altogether wrong. Amy does feel as though she's given up too much to let her father die without a struggle. Besides, she's deeply angry at fate for doing this to Dad and to her life, and she resents her brothers a little for those five years when they stuck her with the most difficult and prolonged period of Mr. Wolter's home care. Randy and Paul, of course, are both aware of her feelings.

But they're missing some important issues that Amy sees clearly. Mr. Wolter did have an unusually deep aversion to the thought of dying—the death of his buddy in combat seemed to have been significant in forming his attitude toward such matters. While many people would see nothing to be gained for Mr. Wolter by even such a minor intervention as a feeding tube, Amy isn't at all sure *he* would see it that way. He certainly never said anything when he could still talk that made her think he'd eventually want to call it quits. In her opinion, her brothers have lost sight of who their father was. They're being guided by their own values concerning what makes a life meaningful instead of by his, and they're protecting their own interests at their dad's expense.

There are, obviously, real issues here between Amy and her brothers, and the moment before death is hardly the time to start sorting them out. People are upset, a little distrustful of each other, and under time pressure. And there's no way to play it safe. Whichever way they go, they run the risk of wronging and harming their father.

Sorting It Out

What should they have done? Well, they *should* have thrashed the matter out long before now. They ought to have realized that the time was bound to come when Mr. Wolter was ripe for a large-scale medical emergency. But it isn't uncommon, or unnatural, for people to put off thinking about a parent's death until they absolutely have to. It's difficult to face up to the possibility of a crisis, and very easy to put off talking about it.

Now, however, time has run out. They have to make some decisions and make them right away. What will that involve?

First, they will have to decide what kinds of concerns it is legitimate to bring to the table. The overt debate between Amy and her brothers has to do with what their father would have wanted in a situation of this kind. Everybody agrees that this is relevant to deciding what to do. But what about the hidden debate—the suspicions they have about one another's feelings? Each side thinks the others are driving their own agenda instead of concentrating on the real question, What is best for Dad? What would he have wanted for himself if only he could think and talk?

We have already pointed out that the needs and values of any one individual, no matter how ill or helpless, should not be allowed to determine how the family lives. Paul's and Randy's concerns about themselves aren't irrelevant to the decision, even if their interests do run counter to their father's. When caregivers pay heavily in time, emotional upheaval, forgone job opportunities, strained relationships, or money, this can't and shouldn't be ignored—not even if the cost to their dad is some months of his life. Mr. Wolter does have a very poor quality of life; he will die soon no matter what they try to do; medical interventions will very likely cause him some discomfort and even flat-out pain; the devotion, time, and energy that's going into his care is forcing his children to skimp—yet again—on other important family functions and personal projects. In loving families such sacrifices can be made happily and willingly during a crisis, but this is no crisis. It's a chronic, slow hemorrhage of resources that has been going on for a decade.

On the other hand, Amy's considerations can't be lightly dismissed, either. In her concern to do what her father would have wished, she isn't merely trying to second-guess what he would have said ten years ago, or what he'd say now. She's not trying to read the mind of a man whose mind is gone. Instead, she's trying to maintain her father's identity by acting for him in ways that say who he is. Now that he is past almost all forms of self-expression, she is trying to keep faith with him by expressing his selfhood for him, not only to her brothers and to the staff in the ICU, but to herself.

Her brothers are right. Much of her passion does flow from "her own issues." That fact, however, does not disqualify her feelings from consideration. Amy has put a tremendous amount of her life into her father's care, and she has done so lovingly. Losing him to death now, when there's still something that can be done to save him, suggests that the life she has struggled so hard and so long to preserve wasn't worth the effort. She rebels at that notion. She knows it *was* worth the effort, and believes that Dad would agree with her if he could.

So, our first decision is that all these concerns belong on the table. What then? How can Mr. Wolter's children have a useful, respectful conversation about end-of-life decision making for him, when the considerations driving them are so different? When they aren't simply trying to decide what would be best for him, but are also trying to figure out what would be best for *themselves,* individually and as a family?

Amy, Randy, and Paul have had practice with this kind of problem. After all, ten years ago they did work out their "shuffling around" arrangement as an attempt to take into account their love for Dad, their own need to have lives not completely taken up by his care, and their respect for his strong aversion to nursing homes. That arrangement, while by no means perfect, proved workable for quite a while. No one burned out completely, and Dad stayed out of a nursing home for seven years. And then, when they all had to bow to the inevitable, they also worked out a routine at Cedarcrest for keeping him as comfortable and happy as possible. Still, the burden wasn't divided equally and Amy is aware of that fact.

Things are even more difficult now. Ten years ago, everyone agreed on the goal: to give Dad as good and independent a life as he could have and by all means to keep him out of nursing homes.

Three years ago, the goal was still to give him as good a life as he could have. What's the goal for now? Are they supposed to keep him alive as long as humanly possible, independent of costs to him or anyone else? Are they supposed to do their best to see that his care goes as he would want it? If the only alternatives are to die now or to lie deeply demented in a nursing home with a tube in his stomach, does it even make sense to talk about what he would want? Isn't it pretty clear he wouldn't want either one?

If you asked Amy to state the goal for now, she'd say it's that everybody continue to affirm clearly and powerfully that their father's life matters. You can't do that, she would say, if you let him die from conditions that medicine might be able to ease. Continuing to care for him is a way of showing the importance of his life overall. People are precious, she reminds her brothers, even when they're a major bother to other people.

Of course he's going to die sometime. We're all going to die sometime, and most men in their mid-eighties who have serious health problems will probably die sometime soon. That in itself is no good reason, argues Amy, to deny him the medical treatment that might postpone death for a while, particularly if the treatment can be provided without causing him great pain or discomfort.

And what about Paul and Randy? Paul doesn't disagree with the goal of saying clearly, in deed as well as word, that Dad's life is just as important as it ever was, even though he is demented. He agrees that their decisions now will say a lot about how much they value their father, and even about how they value the way they have been spending their lives during the past ten years.

However, Paul does want to figure out what Dad's view of further treatment would have been, now that the question is whether to be or not to be. It's all very well to say he wouldn't have jumped at either alternative, but he might have hated one less than the other. Paul thinks he knows which one his dad might have hated less. He wasn't the kind of guy who wanted life at any price so long as he could keep breathing. He took a lot of interest in improving himself and in making a better life for his family. He personally liked an outdoor life—especially if he could go fishing. It's true that he never said anything about refusing life-sustaining treatment. True too that as a volunteer firefighter he had plenty of opportunity to see the impact of high-tech medicine on badly injured people, and he could have said what he thought if he'd had any objections to it. But from his silence it doesn't follow that he thought bare biological life the most important thing in the universe or that it must always take precedence over any other consideration. He never said anything like *that* either.

Paul thinks it's reasonable to see their father's

values as complex, rich, and possibly conflicting. What he would do if he were miraculously restored to health for an hour would probably be to ask his kids what *they* thought was best for him—and for them too. If you ask Paul, Dad's track record in life gives them ample reason to think that the interests of his children were important to him, and that he would take seriously both what his family were facing and what they had already done for him.

Randy has a somewhat different take. He agrees with Amy that if Dad could be helped by something that wouldn't cause him much pain or scare him too much, they'd have to consent to it or they wouldn't be able to live with themselves. He also agrees with her when she says it's too difficult to guess what Dad would want now if only he could still want anything. But Randy thinks the operation to put in the feeding tube will hurt; and that down the road, thumping his chest and shocking him if his heart should stop will hurt; and that most of the other medical interventions that might become necessary will hurt. Maybe none of these things would frighten Dad; maybe he's too far gone for that. But he's also too far gone to be able to tell himself that the pain has a good purpose, or that it won't last long. Randy thinks it's hard to say whether his father can still be terrified, but he knows that the old man becomes agitated when Randy has to move his stiff arm to get his T-shirt on, that he's feeling something unpleasant. He thinks they could spare him more serious pain by letting him go now.

Finally, their discussions helped them come up with some goals they can all live with. They agreed on Amy's goal of acting only in ways that would honor their dad's life. They also agreed that this goal was consistent with not burdening him any more than they could help. They decided they didn't have an obligation to authorize burdensome treatment, and on further reflection they concluded *that* pretty much ruled out any kind of emergency resuscitation. They figured that since there had been no obligation to treat his infection aggressively in the first place, they were ethically safe in refusing the feeding tube now. They agreed not to authorize cardiopulmonary resuscitation (CPR) when Dad's heart stopped, as it surely would in the next few days if he weren't fed.

SECOND THOUGHTS

As the evening went by and the implications of the agreement sank in, Amy started to have some misgivings. Although in his present condition Dad couldn't understand and might be distressed by the care he would need, she never related to her father solely in terms of his present condition. In caring for a badly demented man who now recognized neither her nor himself, she considered herself a character in an ongoing story in which they both had a part.

When she was a newborn, recognizing neither her family nor herself, incontinent, unable to speak, he had changed her diaper and fed her with an eye not only to who she was, but to who she would become. Something of the same thing was happening now, only backward. Just as the future had shaped the relationship Mr. Wolter had with her when she was an infant, so did the past permeate the relationship she had with him now. She wondered if her father—when she thought of him across the full span of his life—would want that life to end just because he couldn't understand what the pain was all about.

Amy's husband, Lewis, had been working the swing shift the night the Wolter children had this discussion. It was late when he got home, but it was soon clear to him that he wouldn't be going to bed for quite a while. Amy was very upset about the way the decision had gone. She was now much less comfortable with what had seemed so reasonable to her earlier in the evening. She was also concerned that if she said anything, her brothers were going to think she had reneged on their agreement.

"Honey, are you sure Gramps would see things the way you do, and not the way Paul and Randy do?" Lewis asked.

"I'm not sure at all. That's the worst part, I

think. What they say seems reasonable, and I can see Dad buying it. But I can also see him feeling about it the way I do. What scares me the most is that my own ideas keep moving around, and I haven't got a clue as to whether that's because I'm starting to see things more clearly, or because I'm just becoming more selfish."

"Hey, you're not becoming more selfish. Nobody who knows you at all could think that—particularly not Gramps. You know what I think? I think Gramps's ideas would keep moving around just like yours do if he were trying to make this decision."

"Maybe . . . but that doesn't make it any easier. I keep flip-flopping, he'd flip-flop too, maybe even Paul and Randy flip-flop a little. The problem is how to stop flopping."

Lewis thought this over for a few seconds. "How did your dad solve problems like this before he got sick? I don't mean about medical care—I know he didn't talk too much about that. But about other important things."

"Well, I remember when he was thinking about giving up firefighting, he and I had a long talk. It was real important to him, but he had gotten the feeling that he was getting too old for the heroic stuff, that he couldn't make the same kind of contribution he used to. We had another long talk when he was first thinking about retiring from his job."

"You were his sounding board, eh?"

"No," she answered slowly. "Not really a sounding board. I was more active than that. Dad tended to be a little . . . I don't know, maybe you'd say indecisive about big decisions like those. I tried to help him know his own mind, but I guess what I really ended up doing was giving him advice. He took it, too, both times."

"You know what I think, Amy? You were helping him to know his own mind at the same time that you were making it up for him. Tell me, were those easy decisions for you?"

Amy smiled and shook her head. "They were godawful. I knew how much those jobs meant to Dad, and I also knew how strongly he felt about having to do a good job at whatever he did. But he was looking to me to help him, so he could stop flip-flopping and make a decision."

"And he trusted you to make a good one, didn't he?"

"I guess so."

"Well, I think he's trusting you now, too. I know this might sound odd, but I think you're making up his mind for him this time, just as much as you ever did. What you decide *is* his decision. That's the way he always did it."

Amy thought about it. "Yeah," she answered slowly. "That's weird but true. I never thought about it that way before. I'll tell you what, though.

I'm still just as far from knowing what to do as I ever was."

"Maybe, but now you know whatever you do decide, that's his decision, too. There isn't much danger that you won't be taking him seriously enough. No more danger than there would be if you had to make a hard decision for yourself."

The immediate effect of Lewis's idea was to help Amy get to sleep. The longer term impact was that she called her brothers the next day and asked if they could get together just one more time to go over the feeding-tube decision.

At that meeting, Amy told her brothers that she had had second thoughts. She still believed it would do more harm than good to pull out all the stops the next time Dad had a medical emergency. But she didn't think that meant they should reject every other kind of life-prolonging care for him. Instead, they should think through each treatment as it came up. In weighing its burdens against its benefits, they should take into account their best sense of what their father might have wanted, of who he was, as well as what his life was like now, and what the implications of such decisions would be for them.

"The big question about the feeding tube, I think, is what is Dad's life going to be like if he gets this procedure done? Is there anything left for him that he might still enjoy? I think there might be. Think how much he used to like to sit in the sun when he was fishing, even if the fish weren't biting. Lots of times he didn't even bait the hook. He just shut his eyes and got blissful—fell asleep half the time. He took real pleasure in that. And you all know how much he likes it when you rub his back with that little wooden back-massager. If he's agitated it calms him right down.

"I think there could still be sensations like that left for Dad. Maybe the feeding tube could give him another few months of feeling the warmth of the sun on his face and a few more nice back rubs. That's not much, I admit, but so far as we know, being dead is even less interesting."

Paul smiled a little at that, as Amy had intended he should. "He'd have to go back to Cedarcrest, you know," he said.

"I know, and I don't like that. But he doesn't know he's in the ICU now and he won't know he's at Cedarcrest. What he will know about is the sun and the back rubs, and we'll all visit him a lot, won't we? We've been so good about this for the past ten years—it can't last much longer. Let's give him this last little bit. Please."

Paul, Randy, and Amy ended up agreeing to authorize the placement of the tube, and at the same time to work out with Mr. Wolter's treatment team a good understanding of the kind of care he'd receive both in the hospital and at Cedarcrest. It was important to all of them that their father not be subjected to any further emergency care—no more ambulances, no more respirators, no CPR—but that his comfort should be a high priority and his life extended as long as it could be without having to do anything that would distress him too much.

And that's largely what happened. The tube was placed, he went back to Cedarcrest, and about two months after that, Mr. Wolter died in his sleep. In the interim, his children and their families had a good chance to say good-bye. Whereas there had been something very indefinite about Gramps's illness before, they all realized now that this was the very last chapter of his life, and they were all happy to have been in on it. Mr. Wolter got a number of very good back rubs. And it was unusually sunny that autumn.

6

Building Bridges

JEANNE QUINN is looking at her pale, red-eyed reflection in the mirror of the ladies' room at Rooney's funeral parlor. It is late in the afternoon, the second day of her husband's wake. She has been playing the grieving but composed widow to perfection—trying hard to make everybody as comfortable as possible in what they must all think of as a "difficult" social situation. Her face is startlingly white above her black dress, and for a moment, she fumbles in her purse for her makeup. But no, she thinks, she'd probably just make matters worse, and anyway, who cares? Not she, certainly, and with this realization, some fortification in her crumbles. She starts to tremble slightly, and knows that if she has to go back into the room where her husband's body is being shown and make polite small talk to a collection of people she

never, ever wants to see again, she'll start screaming at them.

It's better in the smoking lounge, which is blessedly empty. For the first time all day, Jeanne isn't being hovered over by family, friends, or funeral directors. She feels hollowed out, but she's stopped shaking now and is surprised by how clearheaded she is. She's reached some place where she's neither acutely sorrowing nor simply numb, and certain things start to strike her more plainly than they have before.

When she moved out of her last house to her present apartment, Jeanne somehow got stuck carrying a box of books up two flights of stairs. The relief in her arms and back when she could put the box down was inexpressible, but her limbs were like rubber for an hour afterward and then ached for days. Charles's death feels something like that. She's put down a huge burden of responsibility, but carrying it at all took an enormous toll. And she knows she still has to go through the long process of taking stock of her life with her husband—particularly the last seven years, since the time when Charles started becoming a little confused.

But not now—this is no time to start raking all that up. To distract herself, she starts to think about the wake. It's been very well attended. In fact, it's positively full of familiar faces, although many of them are less familiar than they used to be. Jeanne starts to turn over all these people in her mind. Her kids have come up from Kentucky to be there, and some of her grandchildren also made the trip; her annoying sister, his annoying sister, various other friends and relations, old co-workers, people from the old neighborhood. Many of them have practically been strangers since Charles became—you know.

Everyone was on their best funeral behavior that day, though—supportive, loving, full of funny or poignant stories about Charles and what a terrific guy he had been, and all brimming over with admiration for what Jeanne had gone through in caring for him over those last seven years. Initially, surprised by the turnout, Jeanne had felt buoyed up by all the attention. But that quickly turned to a sense of depression, followed by anger. Somehow, the family's big display of support at the wake only showed how thoroughly her husband had been forgotten by his own people when things became difficult. She too has been largely forgotten. She had cast her lot with her husband, and those who shunned him shunned her too.

Almost everybody did show up for the wake, though, and some had even started to reappear during the last few weeks of Charles's life, when rumors started circulating on the family network that he didn't have much time left. Jeanne had gotten ten phone calls and even a couple of visits from people who had been notable only by their absence for as long as five years.

Jeanne's mouth started quivering again. What was *she* supposed to do? She got to her feet, crushed an empty Dixie cup she had been fidgeting with, and rammed it firmly into an ashtray. Where had these people been when she and Charles needed them? What were they doing here now?

There was an urn of hot water in the lounge. Jeanne made herself the day's eleventh cup of tea and returned to the rocker. For some reason the lounge was still empty. All those folks out in the other room were her family, her friends, people who had shared and created a whole life with her. She was over seventy herself, and it wasn't likely that she could trade these people in for a new set at her age. She'd been almost too busy these last few years to know how lonely she was, but now that the big distraction was gone, there was a large and jagged hole in the middle of her life. How could she reach out to her family and friends when they had all acted so disgracefully? Can I possibly build bridges to these people and still keep some shreds of self-respect, she wondered.

Thinking about her own sense of injury brought with it lots of disagreeable feelings—not all of which had to do with her relatives. The nagging sensation, long repressed, that her own care for her husband hadn't been beyond reproach, made its way into her head, and she didn't have the strength to beat it back.

Charles had been reluctant to get any medical

opinion about his growing confusion—which was typical, she thought—and Jeanne had had to push pretty hard to get him to make the rounds of doctors. She couldn't even count the times she told him, "Charles, if you've got Alzheimer's, you've got Alzheimer's. If you don't, you don't. We're both probably worrying ourselves to death for nothing. And if there is something to worry about—well, the diagnosis won't make us any worse off."

But it did. Worry gave way to waves of depression and anger that hit them both at different times and in different ways. The dementia label put a decisive end to the sexual side of their relationship. Jeanne simply couldn't summon up any interest after that, although Charles had been disgustingly interested for quite a long time. Jeanne winced as she remembered some of the bedroom scenes they had had, and how hurt Charles had been when she took over the spare room for her own.

As time went on, the fights about sex stopped, but Charles became much more difficult in other ways—prone to be loud and angry as often as not. But on thinking it over now, she felt uneasy about how willing she'd been to employ hefty doses of drugs to quiet him when he had been obstreperous, even if the drugs did tend to make him dull or half-asleep.

She had also resigned herself back then to the

fact that she'd have to put him in a nursing home at some point. She did her homework, found places that had special Alzheimer's programs, and got him on waiting lists as soon as she could. She managed to find a place for him at the first sign that he was having trouble with his bladder. Charles's sister, Annoying Susan, had objected, saying she thought it was too soon and that Charles would be disoriented, lonely, and frightened. Well, since Susan wasn't paying the piper, she didn't get to call the tune. She and Charles didn't see much of Susan after that.

It was true he seemed homesick and upset at first, although it didn't take him all that long to adjust to his new surroundings at St. Anne's. In fact, he perked up a bit for six months or so, as if he was benefiting from the Dementia Special Care Unit's program. Overall, the three years he spent there seemed to go about as well as they could— which is to say, moderately awful as opposed to unbearable. Surely, he was never neglected in any way or abused. And, she insisted to herself, she had been very much involved with his care from the start.

Actually, it would be more realistic to say that she had been very much involved *at* the start. The staff had gently hinted after the first month that perhaps she was *too* engaged in his care—"It's very understandable, Mrs. Quinn, but there's no need to feel guilty"—and that Charles wasn't being given the best chance to adjust to his new home. That was a hint she took with very little resentment. Maybe, she thought, I took it too easily. Perhaps *all* her disengagement had been too easy. Maybe Charles had gone to the nursing home too early. She could, she knew, have held out longer with him at home if she had really put her mind to it. And maybe, once he was in the home, she had cut back too quickly on her involvement in his day-to-day life.

Not that she didn't visit him religiously every week, if not more often. And it wasn't that she didn't participate in his care when she was there. She read storybooks to him and sang with him, at least while he showed any interest in these activities. After a while, though, it did seem as if she was going because of some kind of vague, social expectation that decent wives visit husbands they've placed in nursing homes, and not because either Charles or she got anything much from the visit. Even when Charles could still go on walks with her, it wasn't really taking a walk together. When she helped him eat, it didn't really seem as if it was Charles she was helping. There came a point when she went to St. Anne's mainly to see the nice people who staffed the nursing home, not to visit her husband. And as the months turned into years, she did get looser about that weekly visit; in fact, she had skipped one of her regular visits on what turned out to be the day he died.

She could almost taste the guilt, but what seemed even more bitter was her awareness that Susan had made one of her own infrequent visits that very day and, therefore, knew Jeanne hadn't been there. Jeanne's attitude toward the rest of the family had hardened pretty early on. She felt it was up to them, not her, to make friendly overtures. She had been the good and dutiful one; they had all been lax. But now she couldn't help thinking she had gotten pretty lax herself. Somehow that didn't make it any easier to deal with her relatives.

What kind of person was she, anyway, that she could be so angry at others for doing what she herself had been tempted to do? No—what she herself had done. Just who had she become over the past decade? Jeanne never used to have such feelings about people. She had thrown herself more thoroughly into her husband's care than anyone else, scorning her relatives and patting herself on the back for doing it, and at the same time she'd been perfectly willing to ignore him—really, it amounted to abandoning him—whenever she had the chance. Talk about hypocrisy! And whatever was she going to do now?

The director of the Dementia Special Care Unit at St. Anne's, Tony Eliot, walked into the lounge and sat down beside her. He hadn't seen Jeanne since the day Charles died. Jeanne had always thought of Tony as a very competent, even creative, sort of person, and anyway, he had kind eyes. He had something else, too—it was his accent, she thought. So many Americans fall for an English accent. Despite Tony's charms, Jeanne had always been a little reserved when she happened to see him at the nursing home, but somehow being here at Rooney's made it easier for her to talk freely. It wasn't too long before she was able to tell him something about her feeling that her family had betrayed her, and that she had betrayed both her husband and herself.

Tony smiled gently and nodded as if he understood. "Why don't you come to our support group meeting at St. Anne's next Saturday?"

Jeanne made herself smaller in her rocker. "I don't think so, Tony, thanks all the same. I never went once the whole time Charles was there. I couldn't see the point of it. What I needed was to *stop* thinking about what was happening—not extra chances to rehash it all. Now that he's dead, what do I want to go back to St. Anne's for? How's *that* going to help me get on with my life?"

"Well," he replied, "I think it could, you know. It's quite possible that seeing how other people have dealt with their problems—their families, their sick relatives, their own guilt feelings—could help you to cope with yours. Besides, I don't see how you'll leave off thinking about things between now and next week."

So the next Saturday afternoon, Jeanne found herself back at St. Anne's, somewhat to her own

amazement. She entered the conference room quietly, a few minutes early, and found a seat at one of a group of four rather rickety folding tables that had been pushed together to accommodate the family members. The other people taking their places seemed to know one another pretty well, but Tony started the meeting by asking everyone to take a turn introducing themselves, and to say a little something about what was on their minds. Jeanne's own participation in this ritual was as brief as she could make it, and the rest of the identity parade was lost on her—she'd never been much good at names, and wasn't getting noticeably better at it as she aged. Besides, she was nervous and skeptical. How could coming to this meeting possibly help?

Jeanne wasn't so distracted, however, that she took no note of what the other people were saying. One rather dramatic-looking woman wearing a lot of silver and turquoise jewelry was talking about how hesitant she had been to take her father to St. Anne's. "Dad was always a very observant Jew. Well, I ask you—Joshua Cantor. You can't get much more Jewish. When it looked as though the only decent place that would take him was Catholic, I was worried. I thought he might think he had died and gone to heaven, only to find out that *they* had been right all along."

Jeanne laughed with the rest of them, albeit a little tremulously. She wiped her eyes and started to pick up the threads of a story being told by a tall black man named Bill.

"Flora was only fifty-four when we got the diagnosis. I'll never forget what happened right after. She didn't say a word in the doctor's office, not a word in the car on the way home. When we got back, she plain ignored all of us—ignored everything, really—for about two weeks. Spent most of her time sitting by herself in a dark room. She fixed herself something to eat most days, or we would have had to make her eat, but that was the only thing she did. She wouldn't talk to us, she wouldn't take any notice of us—she just sat.

"But then she pulled herself out of it. She came out of that room smiling and she looked good—her eyes were livelier and she was holding herself straight again. She said she was starving, so we followed her to the kitchen and watched her fix a big plate of beans and rice. She said she had 'solved' her problem. Here's what she said—she was going to commit suicide."

Nobody moved. Then Tony asked, "How did that make you feel?"

"I was shocked. We were all just appalled. This wasn't any solution. It was just a tragedy piled on top of a tragedy. We all knew she was real depressed, and then we thought that maybe she wasn't thinking straight anymore because of what the disease was doing to her. You know, that she wasn't responsible for her ideas anymore, or else she wouldn't have come up with such a thought.

"But Flora insisted she was anything but depressed. Knowing she didn't have to go through dementia had set her free. She wasn't in the dark anymore—said she felt as though she might actually be able to get some real enjoyment out of life before ending it clean."

"Well, obviously she didn't kill herself," said Tony. "In fact, I stopped by her room this morning and she's doing fine."

"Yes," Bill said, "but in a way, that's what's so awful. For me especially. I couldn't do anything to get her to give up the idea of suicide. To tell you the truth, I ran out of arguments pretty quick. How could I prove to her that what she wanted to do was wrong?

"I did tell her how much it would hurt me and the kids if she died in that way, so violently, before she really had to. But that only went so far with her. She cared about what her death would do to her family, but the way she looked at it, her fate was sealed anyway. I remember she said, 'I've got a very bad, very slow, very terminal disease. It's going to kill me unless I get in there first.'

"She had thought it all through—said that the price to the family if she had to keep on going would also be very high. She felt sure we would all come to realize just why she was doing what she had to do, and we would forgive her."

Marjorie Gibbard, sitting to Bill's left, put her hand on his and said, "I can't blame her for a second, but how awful for you."

"I thought I faced the choice of trying to get her committed or standing by while she took her own life. I couldn't stand either one, so instead I offered Flora a deal. I told her she really didn't want to die now. She was still very healthy, still with it; there was a lot of life left for her. I reminded her that we could do some of the things we had been putting off for a long time, spend more time with the children and the new grandbaby. Then, when things got bad enough that she wasn't having any more fun out of life, if she still wanted to, she could kill herself."

Jeanne was riveted by this story. She had totally forgotten her own worries, and was completely caught up in Bill's. "Is that what happened? She decided to put it off?"

"Not exactly. The idea tempted her, but she was worried that she wouldn't be able to tell when would be the best time to kill herself. If she waited too long, she might get too confused to do it right and she'd maybe end up in a coma or something. She wanted to set some definite date, maybe six months in the future, have a specially good half-year with the family, and then take a lot of sleeping pills.

"So that's how things stood for about five months. Then I played my last card. I reminded her that she was still doing as well as she had been when all this started, and anybody could see it wasn't time yet. I told her that if she'd promise me not to take her own life, I'd do it for her. I gave her my word. So long as she seemed to be having a decent ride, we'd all help her have it to the fullest. When the time came that she needed to go into a nursing home or if she stopped being herself—if she became violent all the time, or abusive, or promiscuous—well, I promised her I wouldn't let her go through that.

"At first, she didn't believe a word I said, though she was touched, you could tell. She wasn't sure I had the guts, and anyway, she didn't think she could ask me to take the risk. But I swore up and down I'd do it. I told her I'd seen how the guarantee that she could escape this thing was giving her strength and peace, and that I didn't want to take that away from her. I said that if loving her as much as I could meant killing her, well, I would love her as much as I could. I said I'd have her with me longer if she trusted me to do it instead of doing it herself." Flora's husband fell silent.

"I'd have said all that to my wife," a burly man in a blue workshirt said abruptly. Marjorie Gibbard looked uneasy.

"Well, it's not so bad now. She doesn't seem too unhappy, really, though she went through some bad patches. I think she likes the things you do here in the special unit, Tony. But I know that if she knew back then what her life would be like now, she'd've been furious that I talked her out of suicide. I couldn't have killed her. I knew that when I promised I would. I knew I had to save her life. But what kind of life did I save for her? I feel as guilty as sin about the whole thing."

The turquoise-jewelry woman, Anne Cantor, jumped on this. "But whose life are we talking about here, anyway? I mean, the Flora who used to hate the idea of being demented is gone now. She's not the Flora who's living here at St. Anne's. The old Flora, the first one I mean, really is dead— at least that's how it seems to me. She just didn't die by taking sleeping pills."

"I've heard that idea before, but hard as I try, I honestly can't see it that way. If I did, what would bring me back here all the time to visit with her? I come because she's my wife and I love her, even though I let her down."

"Right, Bill's right," Barbara Johnson broke in. "When I finally brought my father to St. Anne's, he thought one of the other residents here was my mother. I guess she was flattered or lonely or something—or maybe she thought *he* was *her* husband, I don't know. Anyway, they wanted to move into the same room together, and her family thought that was okay! They said what did it matter now, as long as it made them happier. But it *wasn't* okay. My father adored my mother. He was faithful to her his whole life—faithful to her memory after she died! If I had let him move in with this woman, it would've been like saying I didn't care about who he had been. But it was my job to care. That's just what I'd been doing ever since he became ill—trying to keep alive his connections to who he had been his whole life."

Everybody started talking at once, but the babble died down and Tony seized the chance to say, "Go on, Barbara."

"Well, he made a fuss, but now he doesn't seem to mind. He's not doing very well overall, though. Maybe it would have been better for him, kept him happier, but I just couldn't see it. When we bring people we love here, are we just supposed to forget about who they used to be?"

At the foot of the table a man who'd said his name was Dwayne Bailey looked up from his coffee. He ran his hand vigorously through his hair and asked, "How is being with this woman any different from marrying again?"

"I don't think Dad ever would have married again. I've told you how much he loved my mother. But that's not really the point. It *wasn't* as though he were marrying again. He thought it was my mother. He would have been terribly upset if he had known."

"Would have, maybe, but never could in the real world. Isn't that the point?"

"No, it's not the point at all. I don't believe this stuff about him not being the same person anymore. It's up to me to help him be himself, the person he's always been, because he can't do it on his own now."

Marjorie Gibbard spoke up again. "I don't think it's a matter of who your dad is, but of what's best for him now. Last year there was a badly demented woman here and a rather less confused man who—well, they paired off. Luz and Emmett—remember?" Some of them did. "He asked permission for them to live in the same room, but both their families insisted the staff keep them apart. Emmett actually pined away. Every time I saw him he was sadder and frailer. He died very soon after." There were nods and murmurs. "He died of a broken heart."

Barbara was quiet for a moment. "I still think I did the right thing. I know I have to look out for what my father needs now, and it doesn't bother me very much to play along with some of his delusions. But this one would be right down at his core. If who my father was his whole life means anything, it means that he doesn't treat another woman as if she were my mother."

She blinked the tears out of her eyes. "But I still feel just like Bill does. Guilty as sin. Sometimes I catch myself just wishing he would die, because I don't seem to be able to do anything to keep him in touch with who he was. And *that* makes me feel guilty too."

Jeanne felt brave enough to speak up. "Don't

think it stops after they die," she said. "I never felt so bad about everything as I have since Charles died."

"You mean, there's no relief to look forward to."

"Not so far. I did what I told myself was my very best for Charles, but now I see I was just fooling myself the whole time. And I was mad at everybody else in the family because nobody but me would do their best for him. Mostly, they just dropped us like we were a pair of hot bricks."

The man in the blue shirt, Roy Pyne, frowned at that. "Wait a minute, Jeanne—is that your name, Jeanne? Why did you think you had to do your *very* best for Charles? I mean, why wasn't it enough just to do a good job caring for him?"

"I did do a good job."

"But you feel lousy about it. Why do you feel lousy about doing a good job when we're talking about something incredibly hard to do—something that tears us up emotionally and goes on for years? And you got no help from the family. I think you're hard on yourself. Why isn't doing a good job enough?"

"It certainly doesn't feel like enough. I feel like I let him down, and I don't know how I'm ever going to be able to forgive myself." Jeanne worked to keep her mouth steady.

"Did he make you promise never to put him in a nursing home—stuff like that?"

"No. He was more the 'I don't want to be a burden on my family' type."

"Well, there you are. I mean, if Barbara's right and we're supposed to be faithful to the person we used to know and all, then you ought to be feeling just great about yourself. It seems like you not only did a good job, you did the only kind of job he would have wanted you to do."

"There's another thing that occurs to me about your problem." Amy Wolter spoke quietly. "Your family and friends. Have you thought about what your husband would have felt about them? I mean, would he have felt resentful?"

"No, it took a lot to get him to resent anything. He'd probably have thought they had done about all they could. He certainly wouldn't have wanted me to be mad at everybody. And neither do I, really."

There was a knock on the door, followed by trays of cookies, courtesy of the kitchen. People took advantage of the break. When they had come back to the table, Tony said, "Well, as happens most times we're together, we're hearing a fair amount about people feeling guilty because they aren't sure they've done enough, or done what's right. Who's had any success in trying to deal with their feelings of guilt?"

Dwayne replied first. "It's funny how that works sometimes. I thought I had done a good job being realistic, both about my mother and about myself. I didn't feel guilty, exactly, about the decisions I'd made for Mom, or about how involved I've been in her care. But something was really bothering me, and it came out when I visited her here. I'd be short with her, and I found it very easy to be upset with the staff. Even with you, Tony, as I recall."

"Well, once or twice." Tony smiled.

"I did feel guilty about that. I knew I wasn't behaving very well. But here's the odd part. One evening, I was getting ready to go to sleep, just trying to relax and let my mind go blank, when I had the strangest experience. It was as if I could hear someone speaking to me, saying, 'Let her go.' Just that. 'Let her go.' "

"Weird," said Amy.

"You bet. But I knew right away what the voice was telling me. It wasn't about how my mother was becoming demented and I had to stop pretending she wasn't; I had accepted that. What was getting to me—what I hadn't accepted—was the *way* she was becoming demented. I don't know what I'd been thinking, but I guess I had an image in my head of something like 'dignified dementia,' some picture of the way my mother would do it— the same way she always did everything, with a kind of style. Once I let go of that, I didn't have to be so angry and upset with her anymore. I could just let my mother be who she was. It's helped a lot."

Roy said, "That reminds me of the time I saw the women at the day care center singing 'You Are My Sunshine.' I think I've mentioned that in this group before. Somehow, where—and who—they were didn't seem so terrifying all of a sudden. They were just people with a bad illness that people sometimes get. That helped a lot when I was taking care of my wife. It also helped with my own fears about myself, to tell the truth."

"I've got a story, too," Marjorie Gibbard said, "but it's one I've only been able to tell lately, since Alan's mom has been here at St. Anne's. Since then I've been able to get some distance on the period when she was staying with us—on what it did to our family life as well as the effect it had on each of us personally.

"The thought that seemed to help me the most during the time she was actually living with us had to do with staying connected to myself. I sometimes see myself from the outside, as if I were a dear friend I cared about very deeply. Thinking about myself that way when I'm in trouble helps me to remember that I really like myself, that I'm interested in where I'm going and what I'm doing with my life.

"I've been doing this—I don't know, this connecting—thing for years. But lately it's turned into something different. It sort of expands the connection idea, I guess. Anyway, I was taking a shower one day, right after Alan's mom had moved here, and I was feeling beat and miserable, both because I felt we'd finally failed her in a big way, and because I knew we weren't anywhere near the end of it. I was trying to tap into my 'connection' feeling, when it hit me that there was more than myself here to be connected to. It seemed to me that everything I had been going through, the whole saga of Alan's mom's illness and what it had meant to the family, was immensely *interesting*. Sad, painful, awful, guilt-making, yes—but mainly interesting.

"What the family had been going through together was really fascinating, in a way: figuring out how to help a person we all loved to write the last chapter of her life. Now, maybe it sounds a little cold-blooded to call it interesting—as if I were taking all that pain and putting it under a microscope, but that's not what it's like. It's like the reason the old 'connection' strategy works for me is because I'm absolutely fascinated by what I'm connected *to*. I know I couldn't have felt this way when I was in the middle of the worst of it. But I sort of wish I could have. And I'm glad I'm feeling this way now. It really helps."

"How does it help?" Jeanne asked.

"Well, I guess I should say it helps me. I haven't been able to get Alan to see what I mean, or maybe it just doesn't work for him. My kids understand it better. Anyhow, when I can see my life as bound up in things that really matter, that are enormously—well, interesting—it makes everything easier. It makes me feel as if the pain and guilt I'm suffering are a part of something momentous—not just meaningless, useless misery. My energy is being expended on something fascinating. And I can't tell you how much easier it's been to forgive myself and other people for mistakes and weaknesses since I saw how interesting we all are."

Some people around the table that day—Roy Pyne and Amy Wolter, in particular—found Marjorie's story intriguing; others seemed puzzled by it and pressed Marjorie to explain the full history of the idea, starting with the baby she'd given up for adoption. Even for those who were too caught up in guilt and grief to take the perspective Marjorie was offering, it helped a little to think they might not always feel the way they felt now, and sometime in the future they might be able to look back on this time and say that it was interesting. The group talked on for another hour or so, with old problems being discussed and new stories told, and then everyone went back to their lives, and to their continuing struggle with dementia.

But Jeanne went home with something she hadn't had before. She returned to her third-floor walk-up tired and hungry, but with her head full of what had happened that afternoon at St. Anne's. The story that poor man told about his wife! How absolutely awful. And something Amy had said about Charles not being the kind of person who'd resent the family for dropping out of sight these last few years. She did want to reconnect with her family, but she felt so hurt by them. Maybe if she thought of it as a way of doing what Charles would have wanted, her own pride would be salvaged and she wouldn't feel quite so bad.

Water just about set to boil now, Jeanne noticed. Sauce ready for the microwave. Isn't there some fresher lettuce in here? And what did the woman at St. Anne's mean when she talked about being connected to yourself and interested in what was happening around you? Jeanne didn't know quite what to make of that, but she didn't think she'd forget about it anytime soon. What had happened to her over the past decade *was,* she decided, deeply interesting, and she was very interested in what was going to happen next. She was struck by the positive feelings that came from giving herself permission to think of her life in this way.

Angel hair pasta is ready so fast, that's what's nicest about it, she thought, as she sat down to eat. She poured herself a glass of red wine, lit a candle, and continued to think over the day. Jeanne had been thoroughly uninterested in support groups while Charles was alive. She had always felt she needed whatever space she could get between herself and Charles's illness, and that going to a group to hear other people talk about dementia for hours didn't seem like a very smart way of getting a break. Besides, she didn't think that they'd be dealing with the problems that bothered her the most. Now that Charles was dead, though, and she had seen what went on in the group, she was beginning to change her mind. It did her good to see these people trying hard to stay true to themselves, like when Barbara kept her father from moving in with that woman. That was being true to her own self and true to her father's self, too. And Dwayne, when he told himself to let go of his expectations for how his mother should "do" dementia. What was that, if not a creative way of accepting what couldn't be changed? All of them had been trying to see things clearly, and to help each other do that too. She liked how they gently pushed each other to think about what they were going through. That was what Roy had done for her after she told them how guilty she felt. It wasn't that Jeanne agreed with everything the other people in the group did or said. But she was impressed and comforted by what they were trying to do. She thought she'd go back. Maybe, after she washed up her dishes, she'd give Susan a call.

In this book, we've attempted to offer you who are dealing with the same kind of problems as Jeanne something of the help she's starting to find in the group at St. Anne's. The stories here are not your stories, and the ways in which our characters have thought and acted are not necessarily your ways of

thinking through and acting on the challenges before you. Yet the stories do show people in situations that might seem familiar to you, and we hope
that by reading them you begin to feel less on your
own. We hope they leave you better equipped to
understand and respond to the problems of caring
for a relative suffering from a dementing disease.
Such caring can play havoc with your finances,
your home, your career, your health, and your
feelings. It can also put enormous pressure on
what you may value the most—your sense of integrity and goodness. None of these disturbances
can be eliminated. But by joining your own reflections and hard work with those of others—among
your family, among friends, or even in the pages of
a book—some of them can be made less difficult.
With luck and grace, it may be possible to come
through this time intact—even, perhaps, a little
kinder and wiser.

Appendix

Getting Practical Help: Some Places to Start

OUR STORIES have tried to highlight the many ways in which Alzheimer's challenges our values, and to provide some examples of how people have tried to cope with those challenges. Caregivers may find that their understanding of the nature and importance of safety, or truth-telling, or dignity, or promise-keeping, or of life itself comes under fire as they face dementia in company with their relatives; these have been our chief concerns in this book.

But we don't at all mean to suggest that these are the only kinds of problems family caregivers will face. As we've shown in these stories, caregivers will also need to know how to get hold of good medical services, particularly for diagnostic purposes; Alzheimer's often evades detection for too long. Too, caregivers will need to know who is there to help them as they try to meet the responsibilities of the rest of their lives; where can people turn to find reliable sources of respite? They will often be faced with the need to help a person of fading competence put their financial and legal affairs in order: which lawyers specialize in work of this sort, and how may they be found? In many instances, caregivers will need to consider various forms of assisted living or nursing home placement for their relatives: how may this be done most responsibly and most efficiently? And caregivers will also, quite often, need each other: where are the peer groups that can support caregivers emotionally, be a source of further caregiving stories and tips, and represent the interests of people with dementia and their families to the wider society? In this brief Appendix, we have pulled together addresses, phone numbers, and sites on the internet that caregivers may find useful as they try to meet these needs.

WHAT'S AVAILABLE BY TELEPHONE?

There may be more help than you think, and a good place to start to find out is via the telephone. *Eldercare Locator* is a referral service run by the National Association of Area Agencies on Aging. Callers are asked the name, address, and zip code of the older person, and are then told how to contact Alzheimer's service agencies and other relevant groups in their locality—e.g., their own Area

Agency on Aging or State Unit on Aging. Callers are also directed to the *Alzheimer's Association*. Eldercare Locator can be reached at 1-800-677-1116 on Monday through Friday, from 7 A.M. through 11 P.M. The Alzheimer's Association itself is in Chicago; call either (312) 335-8700 or 1-800-272-3900. There is a special number for the hearing impaired as well: (312) 335-8882. Address for mail: 919 North Michigan Avenue, Suite 1000, Chicago, IL 60611-1676. Another Chicago area–based national organization is the *Alzheimer's Disease and Related Disorder Association*. Their phone number is (874) 933-1000; their address, 4709 Golf Road, Suite 1015, Skokie, IL 60076. The ADRDA coordinates a network of self-support groups with chapters throughout the country; a call to the national office will let you know how to contact the group nearest you.

There is also a phone number for the office of the *National Association of State Units on Aging*—(202) 898-2578—but you can check your own phone listings under "State Government Agencies." The state unit will refer you to your *Area Agency on Aging,* if there is one close to you. Your state unit or area agency may well be a very useful source of referral to many readily accessible resources—support groups, health organizations that specialize in dementia diagnosis, and adult day care services that specialize in Alzheimer's. You might also find it useful to call the *National*

Association of Adult Day Care Services at (202) 479-6974.

The *Alzheimer Society of Canada* is located in Toronto, and can be reached at (416) 925-3552, or, within Canada only, at 1-800-616-8816.

OTHER NUMBERS AND ADDRESSES

- BENJAMIN B. GREENFIELD NATIONAL ALZHEIMER'S LIBRARY AND REFERRAL CENTER, 919 North Michigan Avenue, Suite 1000, Chicago, IL 60611-1676, (312) 335-5767. The Alzheimer's Association numbers—(312) 335-8700 or 1-800-272-3900—can also be used to gain access to the library.

- ALZHEIMER'S DISEASE EDUCATION AND REFERRAL CENTER (ADEAR), National Institute on Aging, P.O. Box 8250, Silver Spring, MD 20907-8250, 1-800-438-4380, Fax (301) 495-3334.

- THE JOSEPH AND KATHLEEN BRYAN ALZHEIMER'S DISEASE RESEARCH CENTER (ADRC), Box 2900, Duke University Medical Center, Durham, NC 27710, (919) 684-6274.

- NATIONAL INSTITUTE ON AGING INFORMATION CENTER, P.O. Box 8057, Gaithersburg, MD 20898-8057, 1-800-222-2225.

HELP ON THE INTERNET

If you have access to the Internet, there is a great deal of information available. For example, the *Alzheimer's Discussion Group* provides a forum for caregivers, researchers, and other interested folks to discuss issues related to Alzheimer's. Sponsored by Washington University's *Alzheimer's Disease Research Center,* the discussion group is offered in both a regular and a digest format. The regular format allows you to participate in discussions, while the digest format may be better if you don't care to be "interactive." To subscribe, e-mail to:

majordomo@wubios.wustl.edu

Messages (other than subscription requests) should be sent to

alzheimer@wubios.wustl.edu

You can also check out their home page at:

http://www.biostat.wustl.edu/alzheimer

The Public Policy Division of the National Alzheimer's Association runs a list which transmits their "Public Policy Alerts" via e-mail. To subscribe, send a message with a subject line reading "E-mail Advocate" and a body stating your e-mail address to:

Jennifer.Zeitzer@alz.org

DIAGNOSTIC RESOURCES

Because getting a diagnosis can often be so difficult, statewide networks of regional diagnostic and assessment centers have been developed in California, Florida, Illinois, Maryland, New Jersey, Ohio, and Pennsylvania; other states may be involved in developing diagnostic networks of their own. We got this list from the very useful *Alzheimer's Day Care: A Basic Guide,* by David A. Lindeman, Nancy H. Corby, Rachel Downing, and Beverly Sanborn. It was published by the Hemisphere Publishing Corporation in 1991. *Alzheimer's Day Care* is particularly rich in addresses for state agencies around the United States supporting Alzheimer's day care and related respite programs with state funds. However, phone numbers and addresses can change relatively quickly; we noticed many alterations as we prepared this appendix.

California, as befits its status as the most populous state, has several Alzheimer's Disease Diagnostic and Treatment Centers:

- UNIVERSITY OF CALIFORNIA AT DAVIS–NORTHERN CALIFORNIA ALZHEIMER'S DISEASE CENTER
Alta Bates Medical Center
2001 Dwight Way
Berkeley, CA 94704
(510) 204-4530

- UNIVERSITY OF CALIFORNIA, DAVIS, ALZHEIMER'S CENTER
  1771 Stockton Boulevard
  Suite 2005
  Sacramento, CA 95816
  (916) 734-5496

- UNIVERSITY OF SOUTHERN CALIFORNIA/ST. BARNABAS ALZHEIMER'S DISEASE DIAGNOSIS AND TREATMENT CENTER
  675 South Carondelet Street
  Los Angeles, CA 90057
  (213) 388-4444

- SOUTHERN CALIFORNIA ALZHEIMER'S DISEASE DIAGNOSTIC AND TREATMENT CENTER
  Rancho Los Amigos Medical Center
  University of Southern California
  12838 Erickson Street, Building 301
  Downey, CA 90242
  (310) 401-8130

- UNIVERSITY OF CALIFORNIA, SAN DIEGO, ALZHEIMER'S RESEARCH CENTER
  9500 Gilman Drive
  La Jolla, CA 92093-0948
  (619) 622-5800

- PROGRAM FOR ALZHEIMER'S DISEASE CARE AND
  EDUCATION (PACE), UNIVERSITY OF CALIFORNIA,
  SAN FRANCISCO
  1350 Seventh Avenue, CSBS-228
  San Francisco, CA 94143-0848
  (415) 476-7605

- STANFORD ALZHEIMER'S DIAGNOSTIC AND RESOURCE
  CENTER
  c/o Palo Alto VAMC
  Psychiatry 116A3
  3801 Miranda Avenue
  Palo Alto, CA 94304
  (415) 493-5000

- UNIVERSITY OF CALIFORNIA, SAN FRANCISCO/FRESNO
  ALZHEIMER'S DISEASE CENTER
  1343 North Wishon Avenue
  Fresno, CA 93728
  (209) 233-3363

- UNIVERSITY OF CALIFORNIA, IRVINE, ALZHEIMER'S
  DISEASE DIAGNOSTIC AND TREATMENT CENTER
  Medical Plaza, Room 1100
  University of California, Irvine
  Irvine, CA 92717-4285
  (714) 824-2382

Florida offers clinics at the following locations:

- MEMORY DISORDERS CLINIC
  12901 Bruce B. Downs Boulevard
  Tampa, FL 33612
  (813) 974-3100

- UNIVERSITY OF MIAMI MEMORY DISORDERS CLINIC
  University of Miami School of Medicine
  1400 N.W. Tenth Avenue, Suite 702
  Miami, FL 33136
  (305) 243-4082

- ALZHEIMER'S AND MEMORY DISORDERS CLINIC
  4300 Alton Road
  Miami Beach, FL 33140
  (305) 674-2543

- DIAGNOSTIC PHYSICIAN'S 1 CLINIC
  P.O. Box 100383
  Gainesville, FL 32610
  (352) 395-0111

Two **Illinois** diagnostic centers:

- ALZHEIMER'S DISEASE AND RELATED DISORDERS
  CENTER
  Southern Illinois University School of Medicine
  P.O. Box 19230
  Springfield, IL 62794-14113
  1-800-342-5748 (within Illinois)
  (217) 782-8249

- RUSH ALZHEIMER'S DISEASE CENTER
  710 South Paulina Street
  Suite 8 North
  Chicago, IL 60612
  (312) 942-4463

Institutes in **New Jersey** include:

- ALZHEIMER'S EVALUATION PROGRAM
  Center for Aging
  42 East Laurel Road
  Suite 3200
  Stratford, NJ 08084-6843
  (609) 566-6843

In **New York,** the diagnostic and treatment centers are called Alzheimer's Disease Assistance Centers (ADACs), and are sprinkled throughout the state:

- ADAC OF LONG ISLAND
  99 South Street
  Suite 106
  Patchogue, NY 11772
  (516) 935-1033

- ADAC OF CENTRAL NEW YORK
  550 Harrison Center
  Suite 120
  Syracuse, NY 13202
  (315) 464-6097

- ADAC OF THE FINGER LAKES
  274 North Goodman Street, Box K3
  Suite 401
  Village Gate
  Rochester, NY 14607
  (716) 442-7319

- ADAC OF NORTH EASTERN NEW YORK
  SUNY at Plattsburgh
  Sibley Hall-227
  101 Broad Street
  Plattsburgh, NY 12901-2681
  (518) 564-3377

- ADAC OF WESTERN NEW YORK
  Deaconess Center
  1001 Humboldt Parkway
  Buffalo, NY 14208
  (716) 886-4400

- ADAC OF BROOKLYN
  370 Lennox Road
  Brooklyn, NY 11226
  (718) 270-2452

- ADAC OF THE HUDSON VALLEY
  Burke Rehabilitation Hospital
  785 Mamaroneck Avenue
  White Plains, NY 10605
  (914) 948-0050, ext. 2375 or 2419

- ADAC OF THE CAPITAL REGION
  2212 Burdette Avenue
  Troy, NY 12180
  (518) 272-1777

Diagnostic resources in **Maryland** vary by region. Central Maryland and the Maryland/Washington corridor have many diagnostic facilities, most located within community hospitals. In western Maryland, contact the Alzheimer's Disease and Related Disorders Program at Washington County Hospital, 322 East Antietam Street, Suite 305, Hagerstown, MD 21740, (301) 582-3080. In eastern Maryland, try the local Alzheimer's Association chapter or a community hospital in Baltimore or Wilmington.

Pennsylvania has twenty comprehensive geriatric assessment programs located throughout the state, offering full programs for memory disorder diagnosis, treatment, and caregiver support. Contact the Project Office of the Alzheimer's Disease Initiative for the Commonwealth of Pennsylvania, 400 Market Street, Rachel Carson State Office Building, Harrisburg, PA 17101-2301, (717) 783-1550.

FURTHER ETHICS RESOURCES

And finally, if you are interested in pursuing in greater depth the kind of ethical questions we've explored here, you might find it helpful to know more about the *Hastings Center,* 255 Elm Road, Briarcliff Manor, NY 10510. The Hastings Center publishes the *Hastings Center Report* six times a year; it is one of the very few publications focusing on ethics which aims to achieve both scholarly excellence and wide accessibility in its articles. Memberships in the Hastings Center, carrying a subscription to the *Report* as well as other benefits, are available for $55 a year ($42 for seniors and full-time students).

Sources and Suggestions

AS WE HAVE ALREADY ACKNOWLEDGED, our greatest help in preparing this book came from the family members who shared their stories with us and helped us to understand what they were going through. We also benefited enormously from our professional consultants. But a third source of help came from other writers' books and articles. We want to acknowledge these writers, and also offer our readers suggestions for further reading.

Three books in particular were useful in the writing of *Alzheimer's: Answers to Hard Questions for Families*. One is *The Caregiver's Guide: Helping Elderly Relatives Cope with Health & Safety Problems*, written by Caroline Rob with the help of Janet Reynolds, and published by Houghton Mifflin in 1991. The second is *Broken Connections*, a book in two parts written by Liduin Souren and Emile Franssen, and published by

222 *Alzheimer's*

Swets and Zeitlinger in 1994. The third is *The Thirty-Six Hour Day,* by Nancy L. Mace and Peter V. Rabins, published by the Johns Hopkins University Press in 1982. *The Thirty-Six Hour Day* is something of a classic in this field, and it is particularly full of interesting (if occasionally controversial) ideas: Roy Pyne in Chapter 3 got the idea for stamping Marie's checks "void" from reading this book.

Regarding the importance of families in helping people form their personalities and hold themselves together as life goes on, we have learned a good deal from Salvador Minuchin's book, *Families & Family Therapy,* published by Harvard University Press in 1974.

The work of Tom Kitwood and his co-workers from the University of Bradford in the United Kingdom has also been very important to us as we thought about the relationship between what happens inside the head of a person suffering from dementia and what happens in their day-to-day surroundings. Kitwood's opinion is that dementia arises both from damage to the brain and from a social environment that is disrespectful to elderly people. Many of his articles have been printed in a journal called *Ageing and Society.* A particularly interesting piece he wrote with Kathleen Bredin, called "Toward a Theory of Dementia Care: Personhood and Well-Being," was published in 1992 in volume 12, pages 269–87, of *Ageing and Society*.

Another article very much worth reading in the same volume of *Ageing and Society* is Steven Sabbat and Rom Harré's "The Construction and Deconstruction of Self in Alzheimer's Disease," which is on pages 443–61. If you're interested in the discussion between Anne and Bill in Chapter 6 about who Flora really is, you will find that Sabbat and Harré say some very useful things. We are also indebted to them for the story of Henry the lawyer, which you read in our Introduction.

We learned a lot about the kind of world confronting Marie, who figures importantly in Chapter 3, from reading Diana Friel McGowin's touching story of her own struggle with dementia, *Living in the Labyrinth,* which was published in 1993 by Elder Books.

We have also drawn heavily on the work of Margaret Urban Walker in preparing this book. We made particular use of two of her essays, both published in *Metaphilosophy*. One is "Moral Luck and the Virtues of Impure Agency," published in 1991 in volume 22, pages 14–27. The other is "Moral Particularity," published in 1987 in volume 18, pages 171–85.

We read Stephen Post's book, *The Moral Challenge of Alzheimer Disease,* in manuscript and found it interesting; Johns Hopkins University Press published it in 1995. Another book you might like is Beverly Coyle's novel about Alzheimer's disease, entitled *In Troubled Waters,* published by Ticknor & Fields in 1993. And a nurse-administrator and family caregiver, Barbara Bridges, has written *Therapeutic Caregiving: A Practical Guide for Caregivers of Persons with Alzheimer's and Other Dementia Causing Diseases,* published in 1995 by BJB Publishers, 16212 Bothell Way S.E., Suite F171, Mill Creek, WA 98012.

We've also used a little of our own earlier work. We first discussed the *Howards End* example from Chapter 5 in an article called "Guided by Intimates," which appeared in the *Hastings Center Report* in 1993, in volume 23, number five, on pages 14–15. We discuss other matters concerning families and caring for aging relatives in the fifth chapter of our book *The Patient in the Family,* published by Routledge in 1995.

THE BEER CAN BY THE HIGHWAY

Books by John A. Kouwenhoven

THE BEER CAN BY THE HIGHWAY
THE COLUMBIA HISTORICAL PORTRAIT OF NEW YORK
MADE IN AMERICA: THE ARTS IN
MODERN CIVILIZATION
ADVENTURES OF AMERICA, 1857–1900

With Others

AMERICAN PANORAMA, *Edited by Eric Larrabee*
CREATING AN INDUSTRIAL CIVILIZATION,
Edited by Eugene Staley

JOHN A. KOUWENHOVEN

The Beer Can
by the Highway

Essays on What's "American"
about America

DOUBLEDAY & COMPANY, INC.
Garden City, New York

Grateful acknowledgment is made for permission to use excerpted material from the following sources:

"Farewell Architecture" reprinted from *Architectural Record,* April 1960. Copyright 1960 by F. W. Dodge Corporation with all rights reserved.

"Whatever Became of Architecture?" published by the Architectural Society of the Rhode Island School of Design, and reprinted with their permission.

"What Is 'American' in Architecture and Design?" revised and expanded from an original article in *Art in America,* Fall 1958.

"Liberal Crafts and Illiberal Arts" revised from a keynote address given at the annual Conference of American Craftsmen and partly published in *Industrial Design,* October 1959.

Designed by Edwin Kaplin

CONTENTS

FOREWORD TO THE READER

THOSE WHO READ THESE ESSAYS in the order in which they are presented will find, I trust, that they build upon one another. They may be read in random order, but I hope they will not be, for I have done my best to write (and rewrite) them in a way which makes each of the later ones evolve from those which precede it.

The first one tries, by indirection, to suggest the limitations of the point of view from which I have looked at the United States. The next two introduce the general question of what is "American" in our civilization and suggest some answers.

The fourth and fifth essays touch upon some of the ways in which education and our ideas of "culture" may unfit us for the "American" world. Then come four essays dealing with the ways in which "American" qualities are expressed (or stifled) in the arts of design, with particular emphasis on architecture, industrial design, and advertising layout.

The final essay, which gathers up threads of idea and attitude from the earlier essays, will, I hope, lead the reader as it did the writer to look with unaccustomed eyes at some contemporary

manifestations of the energies which are likely to shape our future.

J.A.K.

December 20, 1960

Preliminary Glance
at an American Landscape

From the blister-dome of the Wabash Railway's *Blue Bird*, en route from St. Louis to Chicago, the spring landscape of central Illinois is one of wide, level horizons with now and then a clump of leafed-out willows or a brief row of maples or elms which have budded enough to look hazy. It is a land of pale coffee-colored fields, darkened in irregular blotches where cloud shadows lie and in strips where a tractor-drawn disc harrow has recently passed. A lone man driving a tractor is the only human being you are likely to see for miles, but there are many other living things: cattle—black, or black and white, and still winter-fuzzy—standing or lying in the unplowed fields; pigs and sheep whose young scamper away from the fenced railroad track when the train passes, though their elders are accustomed and remain still; and quite often a pheasant, green neck feathers shining in the sun, standing close to the track, always with his back turned to the passing train, looking over his shoulder at it but not otherwise disturbed.

The only city you go through is Decatur, a momentary collection of factories, warehouses, and

handsome grain elevators, and a business district with some stone buildings of modest dimensions. Most of the towns you go through are small and irregularly square, with streets at right angles to the railroad, many of which do not cross the track but stop short at earth mounds partly covered with grass. Each town has a corrugated sheet-metal grain elevator and a Quonset warehouse or two near the wooden station. The houses are wood, with fruit trees blooming in their board-fenced yards. But there are almost no people in sight, just a few cars moving in the streets or parked at the curbs. And in less than a minute you are out on the prairie again.

Occasionally the level fields are studded with shining ponds, and now and then you see small streams whose flashing surfaces are almost flush with the fields they flow through, or shallow gullies banked with tin cans and bottles which glitter in the sun. Running alongside the track all the way, three tiers of shining wires dip from and rise to the crossbars on the telegraph poles—each of the three crossbars with room for ten bright insulators, some missing, leaving gaps like broken rake teeth. Sometimes the ground bordering the track also dips and rises where the right of way has been sliced down to grade through long, flowing swells of land. But the only real break in the general flatness is a huge eroded mesa, man-made from the waste of what may be strip-mining operations, which stretches along

west of the track for miles, somewhere near Red-
dick or Essex judging by the timetable.

Most of the time there is just the wide, flat
landscape of harrow-smoothed earth, ruled into
squares by lines of wire fence strung on thin metal
posts (not split wooden posts, as in New England),
and along the fences there is a fringe of the dry,
blond husks of last year's uncut grass, with now and
then a large, unaccountable sheet of wilted brown
paper caught on the wire barbs. Once in a huge,
immaculate field near Symerton, roughly forty-seven
miles out of Chicago, I saw a rock. It was about
the size and shape of a dented watermelon, but no
one had bothered to move it; the parallel harrow
tracks in the smooth dirt diverged to avoid it, then
came together again.

Once in a while you see white roads taped
across the landscape, and if they cross the track the
diesel honks at them. Once in a while you see a
lonely schoolhouse, usually of wood, with a flag
flying briskly from a pole in front and a yellow bus
standing in the grassless yard. Once in a while a
field is dotted with round metal grain bins with
cone-shaped roofs, looking like a battery of stumpy,
unlaunchable rockets. And once in a while, too, near
one of the clumps of trees, you see a white farm-
house, with red or white barns—big barns, with venti-
lators on their roofs looking like little barns strad-
dling the ridgepoles of the big ones. Near the houses
tall windmills stand on spindly iron legs, mostly with

broken blades in their fans, and almost every farm has a gawky television antenna in the yard as tall as, or taller than, the windmill.

This is a landscape which a century ago looked to a Chicago newspaperman like "the untilled and almost untrodden pastures of God." Standing with a group of excursionists in the middle of the rolling prairies, the reporter, Benjamin F. Taylor, felt as if he were in the center of a tremendous dish.

> Not a tree nor a living thing in sight; not a sign that man had ever been an occupant of the planet . . . The great blue sky was set down exactly upon the edge of the dish, like the cover of a tureen, and there we were, pitifully belittled.

A century later the pastures of God are welltilled and much trodden. The prairie has become, in fact, a technological landscape: subdivided by wire fences, smoothed by tractors, tied to the urbanindustrial world by wires, roads, and rails, and by the invisible pulses felt in the lofty antennas. The height of those antennas measures the strength of the city's pull. As you leave St. Louis they grow taller and taller until, in central Illinois they outtop and almost outnumber the trees. As you approach Chicago they grow shorter until, when you reach the suburban landscape of supermarkets, drive-ins, and rows of little square houses with little square lawns,

they need be only small, solicitous bundles of branching wire rods attached to the house chimneys.

The prairie landscape no longer belittles man. It is still vast, and you see very few people as you watch from a train window. But man's technology has modified everything from the texture of the earth itself to the stance of the pheasants.

This landscape, through which I last traveled three years ago, came freshly to my mind as I began to assemble and revise the essays in this book. It did so, I think, because it embodies a number of the forms and patterns which seem to me to be characteristic of a civilization based as ours is upon a distinctive blend of technology and a somewhat untidy but dynamic form of democracy. And it is with some of these characteristic forms and patterns, and the indigenous energies they express, that these essays are primarily concerned.

There are other American landscapes, some of which embody forms and patterns that seem to have little in common with those of the prairies: the landscape of Maryland's trim and cultivated Eastern Shore; the barbaric splendor of the Southwest's mesas and canyons; the grim and powerful landscape of River Rouge; and—more like the prairies than at first appears—the New York skyline.

The most endearing and comfortable landscape, to me, is in Vermont, where I spend the summers on a farm which lies like a large green saddle blanket on the small of the back of a mountainous ridge along

the western border of the state. Eastward from the farm you can look down into the domesticated Vermont valleys of Pawlet and Dorset, with pasture clearings running well up the enclosing slopes. Westward you look out over a widening, open-ended valley where the tree-hidden village of Rupert lies, where dogs bark distantly in the evening, and where an occasional light blinks through the trees after dark. At the far, open end of the valley the D & H Railroad comes down from the north and curves southward into New York State toward the Hudson and the Susquehanna. You cannot see the trains but when the wind is right—when rain is coming—you can hear the imitation steam-whistle which the railroad, in tune with the new industrial sentimentality, has substituted for barking horns on its diesels. And beyond the valley's open end the continent rolls gently westward through the Mohawk Valley and then invisibly onward past the Great Lakes, lifting easily across the prairies and plains. You can believe that if the atmosphere were glass-clear and the earth did not curve you could see two thirds of the way to the Pacific, for there is nothing high enough to block the view till you come to the Laramie Range and the Big Horns. Closed and friendly to the east, open and inviting to the west, it is a likable landscape.

It is, I suppose, the landscape of this eastward-and-westward-looking Vermont farm, superimposed upon the landscape of New York's skyline, which

controls the point of view from which I have looked at America. But the characteristic landscape of the America I have looked at in these essays seems to me to be the "interminable and stately prairies," as Walt Whitman called them, ruled off by roads and fences into a mathematical grid. They have become, as Whitman thought they would become, the home of "America's distinctive ideas and distinctive realities." They produced Abraham Lincoln and the city of Chicago—both of which are ideas as well as realities and both of which seem to me, at least, to be distinctively American.

The Dispraising
of America*

SOME UN-AMERICAN ADVICE
TO NON-AMERICANS

* This essay grew out of a talk to a group of
foreign students who had come to the United
States on Fulbright scholarships. The group,
which included citizens of several African and
Asian nations as well as some Europeans, were
gathered at the Institute of International Education, on invitation of the Mills College Club
of New York, March 10, 1959.

I IMAGINE THAT one of the most curious, one of the oddest, things that non-Americans notice in America is what might be called the American's self-consciousness about his American-ness. We have been like that for many years—from the very beginning, in fact.

The first published answer to the question "What is an American?" appeared in 1782—just one year after the battle of Yorktown victoriously ended six years of fighting for American independence. The question forms the title of a much-quoted chapter in *Letters from an American Farmer; Describing Certain Provincial Situations, Manners, and Customs, Not Generally Known.*

This book, which first posed the self-conscious "American" question, was written in the English language, for an English audience, by a man born and educated in France, who lived while writing it in New York, but who referred to himself as a Pennsylvanian, and who stopped off in London, to arrange for the book's publication there, while he was on his way back to his native France—whence he would soon return to America as French consul in New

York where (as he told his friend Benjamin Franklin) he enjoyed "The Privileges of double citizenship."

I have deliberately emphasized the mix-up of tradition in Hector St. John de Crèvecoeur's background because I want to suggest that, in a sense, the American self-consciousness about his Americanness is still—as it was in 1782—in great part the result of a feeling or sense of "double citizenship." We Americans are all, in one way or another, aware of a double or bifurcated heritage. The eleventh-generation descendant of immigrants from Holland and the second-generation descendant of immigrants from China are no different in this respect from the eleventh-generation descendant of Negro slaves imported from the Congo. Each of us is conscious of a heritage as an American, and each of us is conscious of another heritage—or, more commonly, of a complex mixture of heritages—from cultures whose values are, in varying degrees, unlike those we have acquired as Americans.

In some sense this is no doubt true of other peoples as well as Americans. One thinks of the Canadians and Australians, for example, or the Liberians or the Israelis. Canada, with its bilingual culture, presents a special problem. It lives with a clear-cut, external duality between English-speaking Canadians and French Canadians, a cleavage which is marked by geographical as well as linguistic boundaries. But in so far as the French Canadian

has been cut off from his French heritage, he was cut off from it by the Englishmen who have become his fellow Canadians, not by an act of his own will. Neither the English-speaking nor the French Canadians, nor the Australians, have voluntarily shattered the continuity of their non-Canadian or non-Australian heritage by an appeal to revolutionary violence, with its inevitable aftermath of resentment and passionate self-assertion.

As for the Liberians and Israelis, however diverse their national origins may be, their motive in immigrating to the countries in which they now live was to re-establish their ties to a heritage even older and more deeply rooted in them than that of the nation from which they came. The immigrant to the United States, however, has always been required (or has deliberately sought) to attach himself to a heritage-in-the-making—a heritage which is not in any sense one to which he is entitled by his ancestry, but one to whose shaping he, as much as (but no more than) anyone else, has the right and duty to contribute.

What James Baldwin, the American novelist, once said of the American Negro can be said with some justice of the white American as well: he arrives at his identity "by virtue of the absoluteness of his estrangement from his past." We Americans do, of course, nourish illusions of recovering the European or African or Asian or American-Indian half of our dual heritage. Some of us even maintain

an illusory sort of psychologically dual citizenship. Such illusions may, indeed, be necessary as long as men are uncertain about the legitimacy of their status, and the American—white or non-white—has never been quite sure what his status is. For we are all, as it were, the younger sons, the disinherited, the bastard offspring of the past. The American estate to which we lay claim is not, and cannot be, ours by right of primogeniture. It is ours only by squatters' right, or by virtue of conquest or piracy or love.

For all these reasons it is true, I think, that the citizens of no other major world power share the special sense of "double citizenship" which from Crèvecoeur's time to ours has made the Americans so self-consciously inquisitive about "What is an American?" A century after Crèvecoeur, Henry James, one of the greatest American novelists, devoted his major energies to the imaginative exploration of the implications of that question, and entitled one of his major novels *The American*. I do not know of (and cannot imagine) any important French author writing a novel called *The Frenchman*, or any Russian writing one called *The Russian*. Our libraries are full of disputatious writings by Americans with titles like *The American Spirit in Art* and *The American Style in Politics*. There *is*, of course, a book called *The Englishness of English Art*—but it was not written by an Englishman, I assure you. Until recently, at least, the English have

confidently known what was English about England and therefore have not had to be self-conscious about it. But the Americans have never been sure what it was to be Americans—which is why, from the beginning, they have asserted so loudly and so inconclusively that they *were* sure. I have a shelfful of books purporting to define the American spirit or the American character and they offer as many different definitions as there are books—all mistaken definitions, too, except one (the one I wrote), and even that one strikes me as slightly tainted by its author's myopia.

Now, the reasons for dwelling at some length on this characteristic in remarks which are addressed to non-Americans is that if you are a visitor or temporary resident in the United States, you probably have some reason to want to understand what the "American spirit" is, or what the "American character's" characteristics are. If you are curious about such things, we will be delighted; and if, when you return to your homes, you write a book about us, telling your countrymen the truth about America, be sure to get the book published in this country, too. It will almost certainly be a best seller—especially if it is very critical and says disagreeable things about the "Snow Queen" frigidity of American women; the low, materialistic interests of American men (and their humble subservience to their womenfolk); the disparity between our professions

of democratic equality and our economic and educational segregation of Negroes; our addiction to comic books and bottled pop; and the rest.

If you write a book giving the lowdown on America from a foreign observer's point of view, you will be in good company. Some very intelligent foreigners have written some very interesting books about us—ranging from the Frenchman De Tocqueville's great work on *Democracy in America,* down through Lord Bryce's study of the *American Commonwealth,* to the Swedish Gunnar Myrdal's *The American Dilemma.* Each of these was and is popular with American readers. But you don't have to be as judicious and encyclopedic as De Tocqueville, Bryce, and Myrdal to be a hit with us. You can be as intemperate as Mrs. Trollope, who flatly told her English countrymen in 1832 that she had discovered the Americans to be horrid: "I do not like their principles," she wrote, "I do not like their manners, I do not like their opinions." And for her courtesy we have rewarded her by buying up unnumbered editions of her book—which is still—after a hundred and twenty years—in print.

The Derogatory Stance

This appetite of ours for comment about us, abusive or judicious, may seem an endearing quality, especially if you are looking forward to getting sub-

stantial royalty checks from an American publisher, but you should be warned that from other points of view it might prove to be a trap.

Put it this way, to start with. Our appetite for criticism and analysis of America by foreigners is an aspect of our self-conscious interest in discovering what "an American" is, and this in turn is a symptom of our not knowing. Since we don't know, and wish very much that we did (our philanthropic foundations spend hundreds of thousands of dollars a year subsidizing studies of precisely this question), we love to listen to anyone who talks as if he knew. If he bases what he says on statistical studies and the paraphernalia of sociological research, so much the better. But if he spins it all out of his head, we don't mind that either.

Being an essentially modest people—or shall I say a people who by education and admonition have been taught that the architecture of Greece, and the Roman code of law, and the painting of Flanders and France, and the ethical wisdom of the Orient, and the poetry and drama of England are unsurpassed and unsurpassable, and that even in technology and science the basic work is all European and we have merely applied the principles ingeniously—being whatever you want to call this, a modest or fundamentally unself-assured people—we find it easier to believe the derogatory things about ourselves than the approving ones. We also find it

easier to say the derogatory things—in fiction, drama, and the expressive arts in general.

Of course there was a time when we could (and did) say the self-approving things. But nobody but an ass could have taken us very seriously in our moods of slapping ourselves on the back, and—as a matter of fact—few people did take it seriously. It was too obviously a kind of whistling in the dark. Not even the writers who "made the eagle scream," as the saying was in the nineteenth century, took themselves seriously; often they were being intentionally funny and fooled nobody except humorless English travelers and some uncommonly stuffy politicians. (I am, of course, oversimplifying here—but it is generally true, I think, that whenever an American says anything very flattering about American civilization, he hastens to counteract it with something unflattering, in order to avoid what he feels would be an air of "I'm better than you," in order to "take himself down a peg.")

The result is that in serious writing about the nature and quality of the American experience, both fiction and non-fiction, whether written by foreigners or by Americans, you are likely to find more that is derogatory than that is approving. And most of what is approving can easily be discounted as ignorant, or superficial, or mere high spirits.

Furthermore—and this is the root of the difficulty, if one is really intent upon learning what

America means—it is very easy to mistake the significance of the literature which criticizes or rejects American culture for its bourgeois values, its materialism, its complacency, and so on. We are all quite likely to take such criticism at its face value, and thereby miss the point. We are likely either to praise it for its success in embodying values "superior" to America's standardized middle-class mediocrity, or, if we are in a chauvinistic or jingoistic mood, to damn it out of hand for its wrongheadedness.

The significance of a novel like Sinclair Lewis's *Babbitt* is, I believe, missed if you conclude from it either that Lewis was "un-American" because he disapproved of businessmen like Babbitt or that his book represents a set of values "superior" to (and therefore not characteristic of) the values of the civilization men like Babbitt had created in America. For Lewis was not writing as one who has descended from a "higher" plane to observe our civilization. He writes as one of us, who has seen—from a perspective which he assumes his fellow Americans can share—the inadequacies, the forlorn limitations of certain aspects of American life—aspects which his readers will reject just as he does. And of course he was right. His novel was a great popular success. His readers, most of whom were in business or commerce, saw in Babbitt some of the very things that they saw in themselves, and toward which they felt, like

Lewis, an odd mixture of sardonic amusement and of loyalty.

What I am trying to suggest is that, if a foreign reader concluded, from the quality of photographic, tape-recorded reality which Lewis's technique imparts to his novel, that Babbitt was the typical American businessman of the 1920's—and if he further concluded that, since American civilization is a business civilization, he could draw from the novel some conclusions about the inadequacies and forlorn limitations of the civilization itself, he would have run a serious risk. Hitler and his cohorts took such a risk, gambling that a nation of Babbitts would not rise to the challenge of Nazi domination of Europe. The leaders of other nations may make a similar mistake if they get the impression from our current non-fiction that we are a nation of juvenile delinquents or if they conclude from our young poets and novelists that our young people are beatniks. For Jack Kerouac and Ginsberg, like Lewis and Mencken in the twenties, do not quite signify what they appear to be saying. Their significance, I think, is that they are witnesses to the basic and neverceasing drive within our culture to lift itself, to be dissatisfied with its limitations, to try—at whatever cost in self-distrust or self-reproach—to discover what, indeed, is an American.

Citizens of a New World

I am afraid I am beginning to sound apocalyptic, as if, like the cheap politician whom the nineteenth-century humorists burlesqued, I were about to make the American eagle scream. I hope that is not what I am about to do.

For what interests me about American civilization is that it is not—even in name—the civilization of the United States. As that name "American" suggests, it is something whose relevance is not confined in political boundaries. I know that we use it that way some of the time. I know that our neighbors in Latin America sometimes are hurt by what they assume to be our arrogance in speaking of ourselves as Americans; for geographically, they are as much Americans as we who live in the United States. But I like to think that at least some of the time we know this as well as they do, and that when we call ourselves Americans we are not implying that they are *not* Americans, but are—on the contrary—thinking of ourselves not merely as citizens of the United States but as people living in a New World. For in a very real sense we, like all people whose lives have felt the impact of the twin energies of democracy and technology, *are* living in a New World—not merely the hemispheric New World of the geographers, but the New World which the great seventeenth-century English physician, Sir Thomas

Browne, called "the America and untravelled parts of truth." Everyone who lives in *this* America, in *this* new and untraveled world, is as much concerned as are those of us who live in the United States to discover "What is an American?"

I am sure that I forget from time to time, as most of my fellow citizens forget, that this New World is not coextensive with my nation, or—more provincial still—with my precinct. I know that United States foreign policy is often not synonymous with a policy which would be genuinely American in the sense of that word I have tried to suggest. But our tendency to behave, much of the time, as citizens of the United States is as human and natural as it is for people in other lands to behave as citizens of Ghana or India or France. We cannot ignore, nor should non-Americans who wish to understand us ignore, the national heritage of the United States and the privileges and obligations of its citizens. But if I am not mistaken what we all really want to know is what Crèvecoeur wanted to know a century and three quarters ago: what is an American? And that question can be answered, I think, only when we discover that non-geographical "America" which is, in fact, the community in whose citizenship all our bifurcated heritages, our dual citizenships, are ultimately involved. We shall know "what is an American," I suspect, only when we know who is fit to be a citizen of the New World to whose dynamics and energies the United States has made large con-

tributions, but which is being shaped by people in all lands where the influence of modern technology, and of a democratic faith in man's unexplored potentialities, have been felt. For America, in this sense, is still in the making—is still the New World to which mankind has for so many centuries been adventuring.

What's "American" about America*

* The first version of this essay was given as a
lecture at the University of Colorado, August 3,
1954, and published in the *Colorado Quarterly*,
Winter 1955. Later versions were read at Smith
College and at the Columbia University Seminar on American Civilization. The present version is revised from one published in *Harper's
Magazine*, July 1956.

THE DISCOVERY OF AMERICA has never been a more popular pastime than it is today. Scarcely a week goes by without someone's publishing a new book of travels in the bright continent. Magazines here and abroad provide a steady flow of articles by journalists, historians, sociologists, and philosophers who want to explain the United States to themselves, or to itself, or to others.

The discoverers of America have, of course, been describing their experiences ever since Captain John Smith wrote his first book about America almost three hundred and fifty years ago. But as Smith himself noted, not everyone "who hath bin at Virginia, understandeth or knows what Virginia is." Indeed, just a few years ago the Carnegie Corporation, which supports a number of college programs in American Studies, entitled its quarterly report "Who Knows America?" and went on to imply that nobody does, not even "our lawmakers, journalists, civic leaders, diplomats, teachers, and others."

There is, of course, the possibility that some of the writers who have explored, vicariously or in person, this country's past and present may have come

to understand or know what America really is. But how is the lay inquirer to judge which accounts to trust? Especially since most of the explorers seem to have found not one but two or more antipodal and irreconcilable Americas. The Americans, we are convincingly told, are the most materialistic of peoples, and, on the other hand, they are the most idealistic; the most revolutionary, and, conversely, the most conservative; the most rampantly individualistic, and, simultaneously, the most gregarious and herdlike; the most irreverent toward their elders, and, contrariwise, the most abject worshipers of "Mom." They have an unbridled admiration of everything big, from bulldozers to bosoms; and they are in love with everything diminutive, from the "small hotel" in the song to the "little woman" in the kitchen.

Maybe, as Henry James thought when he wrote *The American Scene,* it is simply that the country is "too large for any human convenience," too diverse in geography and in blood strains to make sense as any sort of unit. Whatever the reason, the conflicting evidence turns up wherever you look, and the observer has to content himself with some sort of pluralistic conception. The philosopher Santayana's way out was to say that the American mind was split in half, one half symbolized by the skyscraper, the other by neat reproductions of Colonial mansions (with surreptitious modern conveniences). "The American will," he concluded, "in-

habits the skyscraper; the American intellect inherits the Colonial mansion." Mark Twain also defined the split in architectural terms, but more succinctly: American houses, he said, had Queen Anne fronts and Mary Ann behinds.

And yet, for all the contrarieties, there remains something which I think we all feel to be distinctively American, some quality or characteristic underlying the polarities which—as Henry James himself went on to say—makes the American way of doing things differ more from any other nation's way than the ways of any two other Western nations differ from each other.

I am aware of the risks in generalizing. And yet it would be silly, I am convinced, to assert that there are not certain things which are more American than others. Take the New York City skyline, for example—that ragged man-made Sierra at the eastern edge of the continent. Clearly, in the minds of immigrants and returning travelers, in the iconography of the admen who use it as a backdrop for the bourbon and airplane luggage they are selling, in the eyes of poets and of military strategists, it is one of the prime American symbols.

Let me start, then, with the Manhattan skyline and list a few things which occur to me as distinctively American. Then, when we have the list, let us see what, if anything, these things have in common. Here are a dozen items to consider:

1. The Manhattan skyline
2. The gridiron town plan
3. The skyscraper
4. The Model-T Ford
5. Jazz
6. The Constitution
7. Mark Twain's writing
8. Whitman's *Leaves of Grass*
9. Comic strips
10. Soap operas
11. Assembly-line production
12. Chewing gum

Here we have a round dozen artifacts which are, it seems to me, recognizably American, not likely to have been produced elsewhere. Granted that some of us take more pleasure in some of them than in others—that many people prefer soap opera to *Leaves of Grass* while others think Mark Twain's storytelling is less offensive than chewing gum—all twelve items are, I believe, widely held to be indigenous to our culture. The fact that many people in other lands like them too, and that some of them are nearly as acceptable overseas as they are here at home, does not in any way detract from their obviously American character. It merely serves to remind us that to be American does not mean to be inhuman—a fact which, in certain moods of self-criticism, we are inclined to forget.

What, then, is the "American" quality which these dozen items share? And what can that quality tell us about the character of our culture, about the nature of our civilization?

Skylines and Skyscrapers

Those engaged in discovering America often begin by discovering the Manhattan skyline, and here as well as elsewhere they discover apparently irreconcilable opposites. They notice at once that it doesn't make any sense, in human or aesthetic terms. It is the product of insane politics, greed, competitive ostentation, megalomania, the worship of false gods. Its by-products, in turn, are traffic jams, bad ventilation, noise, and all the other ills that metropolitan flesh is heir to. And the net result is, illogically enough, one of the most exaltedly beautiful things man has ever made.

Perhaps this paradoxical result will be less bewildering if we look for a moment at the formal and structural principles involved in the skyline. It may be helpful to consider the skyline as we might consider a lyric poem, or a novel, if we were trying to analyze its aesthetic quality.

Looked at in this way, it is clear that the total effect which we call "the Manhattan skyline" is made up of almost innumerable buildings, each in competition (for height, or glamour, or efficiency, or

respectability) with all of the others. Each goes its own way, as it were, in a carnival of rugged architectural individualism. And yet—as witness the universal feeling of exaltation and aspiration which the skyline as a whole evokes—out of this irrational, unplanned, and often infuriating chaos, an unforeseen unity has evolved. No building ever built in New York was placed where it was, or shaped as it was, because it would contribute to the aesthetic effect of the skyline—lifting it here, giving it mass there, or lending a needed emphasis. Each was built, all those now under construction are being built, with no thought for their subordination to any over-all effect.

What, then, makes possible the fluid and ever-changing unity which does, in fact, exist? Quite simply, there are two things, both simple in themselves, which do the job. If they were not simple, they would not work; but they are, and they do.

One is the gridiron pattern of the city's streets —the same basic pattern which accounts for Denver, Houston, Little Rock, Birmingham, and almost any American town you can name, and the same pattern which, in the form of square townships, sections, and quarter sections, was imposed by the Ordinance of 1785 on an almost continental scale as what Wolfgang Langewiesche has called "a diagram of the idea of the Social Contract," a blueprint for a future society in which men would live each in his

own domain, free and equal, each man's domain clearly divided from his neighbor's.

Whatever its shortcomings when compared with the "discontinuous patterns" of modern planned communities, this artificial geometric grid—imposed upon the land without regard to contours or any preconceived pattern of social zoning—had at least the quality of rational simplicity. The section lines, along which roads and fences run due north-south and due east-west, and which are so clearly visible from a plane over most of the U.S.A., make most of the nation exactly what an airplane pilot wants country to be: graph paper. As Langewiesche, the pilot, has said: "You can time your [plane's] shadow with a stop-watch across two lines, and get your exact speed. You can head the airplane down a section line and check your compass. But you hardly need a compass. You simply draw your course on the map and see what angle it makes. Then you cross the sections at the same angle. You can't miss. If you want to go exactly west, you get on a fence and follow it." And this simple gridiron pattern, mimicked in the city's streets, horizontally controls the spacing and arrangement of the isolated rectangular shafts which go to make up the skyline.

The other thing which holds the skyline's diversity together is the structural principle of the skyscraper. When we think of individual buildings, we tend to think of details of texture, color, and form, of surface ornamentation or the lack of it. But

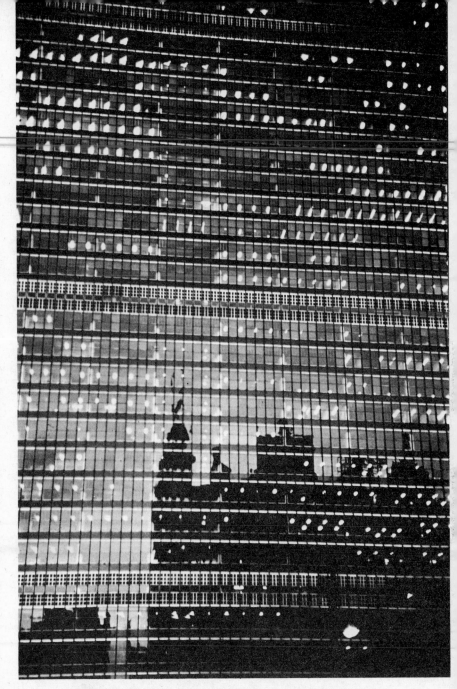

A New York Skyline Reflected in the Façade of the United Nations Building. (Black and white print from a color transparency photographed by Ernst Haas, courtesy of Magnum Photos.)

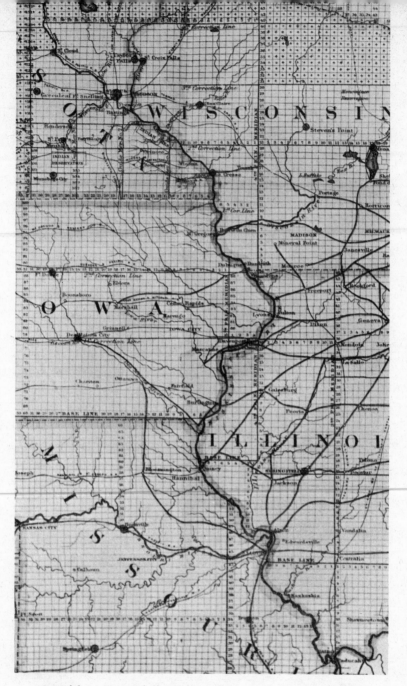

Detail from "Map of the United States and Territories. Showing
the Extent of Public Surveys," Theodore Franks, draughtsman,
1866. From *Report of the Commissioner of the General Land
Office for the Year 1866,* Washington, 1867.

as elements in Manhattan's skyline, these things are of little consequence. What matters there is the vertical thrust, the motion upward; and that is the product of cage, or skeleton, construction in steel— a system of construction which is, in effect, merely a three-dimensional variant of the gridiron street plan, extending vertically instead of horizontally.

The aesthetics of cage, or skeleton, construction have never been fully analyzed, nor am I equipped to analyze them. But as a lay observer, I am struck by fundamental differences between the effect created by height in the RCA building at Rockefeller Center, for example, and the effect created by height in Chartres cathedral or in Giotto's campanile. In both the latter (as in all the great architecture of the past) proportion and symmetry, the relation of height to width, are constituent to the effect. One can say of a Gothic cathedral, this tower is too high; of a Romanesque dome, this is top-heavy. But there is nothing inherent in cage construction to invite such judgments. A true skyscraper like the RCA building could be eighteen or twenty stories taller, or ten or a dozen stories shorter, without changing its essential aesthetic effect. Once steel cage construction has passed a certain height, the effect of transactive upward motion has been established; from there on, the point at which you cut it off is arbitrary and makes no difference.

Those who are familiar with the history of the skyscraper will remember how slowly this fact was

realized. Even Louis Sullivan—greatest of the early skyscraper architects—thought in terms of having to close off and climax the upward motion of the tall building with an "attic" or cornice which should be, in its outward expression, "specific and conclusive." His lesser contemporaries worked for years on the blind assumption that the proportion and symmetry of masonry architecture must be preserved in the new technique. If with the steel cage one could go higher than with load-bearing masonry walls, the old aesthetic effects could be counterfeited by dressing the façade as if one or more buildings had been piled on top of another—each retaining the illusion of being complete in itself. You can still see such buildings in New York: the first five stories perhaps a Greco-Roman temple, the next ten a neuter warehouse, and the final five or six an Aztec pyramid. That Aztec pyramid is simply a cheap and thoughtless equivalent of the more subtle Sullivan cornice. Both structures attempt to close and climax the upward thrust, to provide an effect similar to that of the *Katharsis* of Greek tragedy.

But the logic of cage construction requires no such climax. It has less to do with the inner logic of masonry forms than with that of the old Globe-Wernicke sectional bookcases, whose interchangeable units (with glass-flap fronts) anticipated by fifty years the modular unit systems of so-called modern furniture. Those bookcases were advertised in the nineties as "always complete but never fin-

ished"—a phrase which could with equal propriety have been applied to the Model-T Ford. Many of us remember with affection that admirably simple mechanism, forever susceptible to added gadgets or improved parts, each of which was interchangeable with what you already had.

Here, then, are the two things which serve to tie together the otherwise irrelevant components of the Manhattan skyline: the gridiron ground plan and the three-dimensional vertical grid of steel cage construction. And both of these are closely related to one another. Both are composed of simple and infinitely repeatable units.

The Structure of Jazz

It was the French architect, Le Corbusier, who described New York's skyline as "hot jazz in stone and steel." At first glance this may sound as if it were merely a slick updating of Schelling's "Architecture . . . is frozen music," but it is more than that if one thinks in terms of the structural principles we have been discussing and the structural principles of jazz.

Let me begin by making clear that I am using the term jazz in its broadest significant application. There are circumstances in which it is important to define the term with considerable precision, as when you are involved in discussion with a disciple of one of the many cults, orthodox or progressive, which

devote themselves to some particular subspecies of jazz. But in our present context we need to focus upon what all the subspecies (Dixieland, Swing, Bop, or Progressive Jazz) have in common; in other words, we must neglect the by no means uninteresting qualities differentiating one from another, since it is what they have in common which can tell us most about the civilization which produced them.

There is no definition of jazz, academic or otherwise, which does not acknowledge that its essential ingredient is a particular kind of rhythm. Improvisation is also frequently mentioned as an essential; but even if it were true that jazz always involves improvisation, that would not distinguish it from a good deal of Western European music of the past. It is the distinctive rhythm which differentiates all types of jazz from all other music and which gives to all of its types a basic family resemblance.

It is not easy to define that distinctive rhythm. Winthrop Sargeant has described it as the product of two superimposed devices: syncopation and polyrhythm, both of which have the effect of constantly upsetting rhythmical expectations. Andre Hodeir, in his analytical study, *Jazz: Its Evolution and Essence,* speaks of "an alternation of syncopations and notes played on the beat," which "gives rise to a kind of expectation that is one of jazz's subtlest effects."

As you can readily hear, if you listen to any

jazz performance (whether of the Louis Armstrong, Benny Goodman, or Dave Brubeck variety), the rhythmical effect depends upon there being a clearly defined basic rhythmic pattern to enforce the expectations which are to be upset. That basic pattern is the 4/4 or 2/4 beat underlying all jazz. Hence the importance of the percussive instruments in jazz: the drums, the guitar or banjo, the bull fiddle, the piano. Hence too the insistent thump, thump, thump, thump which is so boring when you only half-hear jazz—either because you are too far away, across the lake or in the next room, or simply because you will not listen attentively. But hence also the delight, the subtle effects good jazz provides as the melodic phrases evade, anticipate, and return to, and then again evade the steady basic four-beat pulse which persists, implicitly or explicitly, throughout the performance.

In other words, the structure of a jazz performance is, like that of the New York skyline, a tension of cross-purposes. In jazz at its characteristic best, each player seems to be—and has the sense of being—on his own. Each goes his own way, inventing rhythmic and melodic patterns which, superficially, seem to have as little relevance to one another as the United Nations building does to the Empire State. And yet the outcome is a dazzlingly precise creative unity.

In jazz that unity of effect is, of course, the result of the very thing each of the players is flout-

ing: namely, the basic 4/4 beat—that simple rhythmic gridiron of identical and infinitely extendible units which holds the performance together. As Louis Armstrong once wrote, you would expect that if every man in a band "had his own way and could play as he wanted, all you would get would be a lot of jumbled-up, crazy noise." But, as he goes on to say, that does not happen, because the players know "by ear and sheer musical instinct" just when to leave the underlying pattern and when to get back on it.

What it adds up to, as I have argued elsewhere, is that jazz is the first art form to give full expression to Emerson's ideal of a union which is perfect only "when all the uniters are isolated." That Emerson's ideal is deeply rooted in our national experience need not be argued. Frederick Jackson Turner quotes a letter written by a frontier settler to friends back East, which in simple, unself-conscious words expresses the same reconciling of opposites. "It is a universal rule here," the frontiersman wrote, "to help one another, each one keeping an eye single to his own business."

One need only remember that the Constitution itself, by providing for a federation of separate units, became the infinitely extendible framework for the process of reconciling liberty and unity over vast areas and conflicting interests. Its seven brief articles, providing for checks and balances between interests, classes, and branches of the government, es-

tablish, in effect, the underlying beat which gives momentum and direction to a political process Richard Hofstadter has called "a harmonious system of mutual frustration"—a description that fits a jazz performance as well as it fits our politics.

The aesthetic effects of jazz, as Winthrop Sargeant long ago suggested, have as little to do with symmetry and proportion as have those of a skyscraper. Like the skyscraper, the total jazz performance does not build to an organically required climax; it can simply cease. The "piece" which the musicians are playing may, and often does, have a rudimentary Aristotelian pattern of beginning, middle, and end; but the jazz performance need not. In traditional Western European music, themes are developed. In jazz they are toyed with and dismantled. There is no inherent reason why the jazz performance should not continue for another 12 or 16 or 24 or 32 measures (for these are the rhythmic cages in jazz corresponding to the cages of a steel skeleton in architecture). As in the skyscraper, the aesthetic effect is one of motion, in this case horizontal rather than vertical.

Jazz rhythms create what can only be called momentum. When the rhythm of one voice (say the trumpet, off on a rhythmic and melodic excursion) lags behind the underlying beat, its four-beat measure carries over beyond the end of the underlying beat's measure into the succeeding one, which

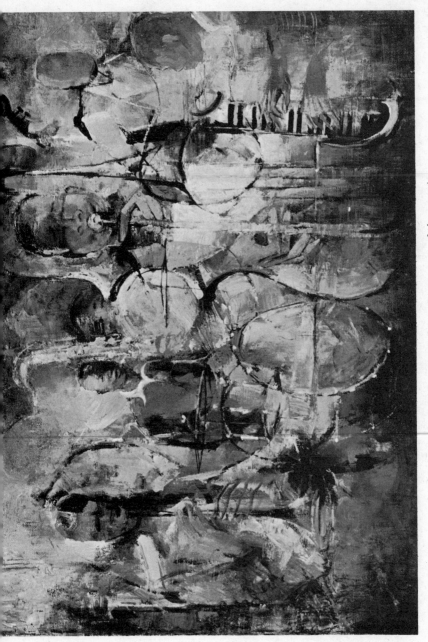

From a painting by Jay Robinson (courtesy of the artist).

has already begun. Conversely, when the trumpet anticipates the beat, it starts a new measure before the steady underlying beat has ended one. And the result is an exhilarating forward motion which the jazz trumpeter Wingy Manone once described as "feeling an increase in tempo though you're still playing at the same tempo." Hence the importance in jazz of timing, and hence the delight and amusement of the so-called "break," in which the basic 4/4 beat ceases and a soloist goes off on a flight of fancy which nevertheless comes back surprisingly and unerringly to encounter the beat precisely where it would have been if it had kept going.

Once the momentum is established, it can continue until—after an interval dictated by some such external factor as the conventional length of phonograph records or the endurance of dancers—it stops. ("No stopping," as the signs on the thruways and parkways have it, "except for repairs.") And as if to guard against any Aristotelian misconceptions about an end, it is likely to stop on an unresolved chord, so that harmonically, as well as rhythmically, everything is left up in the air. Even the various coda-like devices employed by jazz performers at dances, such as the corny old "without a shirt" phrase of blessed memory, are often harmonically unresolved. They are merely conventional ways of saying "we quit," not, like Beethoven's insistent codas, ways of saying, "There now; that ties off all the loose ends;

I'm going to stop now; done; finished; concluded; signed, sealed, delivered."

We think of jazz as a twentieth-century phenomenon, and it is true that it did not emerge as a national music until after the First World War. But there are close (and unexplored) analogies between jazz and other forms of popular arts which have deep roots in our national life. One is the nineteenth-century minstrel show. Constance Rourke gives a vivid description of it in her classic work on *American Humor:*

> Endmen and interlocutors spun out their talk with an air of improvisation. . . . In the dancing a strong individualism appeared, and the single dancer might perform his feats on a peck measure, and dancers might be matched against each other with high careerings which belonged to each one alone; but these excursions were caught within the broad effect. Beneath them all ran the deep insurgence of the Negro choruses . . . and the choral dancing of the walk-around made a resonant primitive groundwork.

Here we have several analogies with the structure of jazz—especially the improvisatory manner and the individual flights of fancy and fantasy held together by a rhythmic groundwork (the 4/4 beat of the walk-around). And there are other ways in which jazz is related to the minstrel show. The min-

strel characters—Jim Crow, Zip Coon, Dan Tucker—
were blackface creations, and many jazz musicians,
both white and Negro, perpetuate the atmosphere
of burnt-cork masquerade.

Related to these analogies are those between
the form of jazz and the form of the humorous monologue, the dominant form in the tradition of American humor, from Seba Smith's Mayor Jack Downing
to Mark Twain and Mr. Dooley and on down to the
TV and night-club entertainers of our own time. In
these humorous monologues the apparent "subject"
is of as little importance as is the tune from which
a jazz performance takes off. It is the "talking
around" the subject without hitting it, the digress-
ing and ramifying, which matters.

Twain and Whitman

Since Mark Twain is the acknowledged master
of the humorous monologue in our literature, let us
look at an example of his work. His writing was, of
course, very largely the product of oral influences.
He was a born storyteller, and he always insisted
that the oral form of the humorous story was high
art. Its essential tool (or weapon), he said, is the
pause—which is to say, timing. "If the pause is too
long the impressive point is passed," he wrote, "and
the audience have had time to divine that a surprise
is intended—and then you can't surprise them, of

course." In other words, he saw the pause as a device for upsetting expectations, like the jazz "break."

Mark, as you know, was by no means a formal perfectionist. In fact he took delight in being irreverent about literary form. Take, for example, his account of the way *Pudd'nhead Wilson* came into being. It started out to be a story called "Those Extraordinary Twins," about a youthful freak consisting, he said, of "a combination consisting of two heads and four arms joined to a single body and a single pair of legs—and I thought I would write an extravagantly fantastic little story with this freak of nature for hero—or heroes—a silly young Miss [named Rowena] for heroine, and two old ladies and two boys for the minor parts."

But as he got writing the tale, it kept spreading along and other people began intruding themselves—among them Pudd'nhead, and a woman named Roxana, and a young fellow named Tom Driscoll, who before the book was half finished had taken things almost entirely into their own hands and were "working the whole tale as a private venture of their own."

From this point, I want to quote Mark directly, because in the process of making fun of fiction's formal conventions he employs a technique which is the verbal equivalent of the jazz "break"—a technique of which he was a master.

When the book was finished and I came to
look round to see what had become of the team
I had originally started out with—Aunt Patsy
Cooper, Aunt Betsy Hale, the two boys, and
Rowena the light-weight heroine—they were nowhere to be seen; they had disappeared from
the story some time or other. I hunted about
and found them—found them stranded, idle,
forgotten, and permanently useless. It was very
awkward. It was awkward all around, but more
particularly in the case of Rowena, because there
was a love match on, between her and one of
the twins that constituted the freak, and I had
worked it up to a blistering heat and thrown in
a quite dramatic love quarrel, [now watch Mark
take off like a jazz trumpeter flying off on his
own in a fantastic break] wherein Rowena
scathingly denounced her betrothed for getting
drunk, and scoffed at his explanation of how it
had happened, and wouldn't listen to it, and
had driven him from her in the usual "forever"
way; and now here she sat crying and broken-
hearted; for she had found that he had spoken
only the truth; that it was not he, but the other
half of the freak that had drunk the liquor that
made him drunk; that her half was a prohibi-
tionist and had never drunk a drop in his life,
and although tight as a brick three days in the
week, was wholly innocent of blame; and indeed, when sober, was constantly doing all he
could to reform his brother, the other half, who

never got any satisfaction out of drinking, anyway, because liquor never affected him. [Now
he's going to get back on the basic beat again.]
Yes, here she was, stranded with that deep in-
justice of hers torturing her poor torn heart.

Mark didn't know what to do with her. He couldn't
just leave her there, of course, after making such a
to-do over her; he'd have to account to the reader
for her somehow. So he finally decided that all he
could do was "give her the grand bounce." It
grieved him, because he'd come to like her after a
fashion, "notwithstanding she was such an ass and
said such stupid, irritating things and was so nause-
atingly sentimental"; but it had to be done. So he
started Chapter Seventeen with: "Rowena went out
in the back yard after supper to see the fireworks
and fell down the well and got drowned."

It seemed abrupt [Mark went on], but I
thought maybe the reader wouldn't notice it,
because I changed the subject right away to
something else. Anyway it loosened up Rowena
from where she was stuck and got her out of the
way, and that was the main thing. It seemed a
prompt good way of weeding out people that
had got stalled, and a plenty good enough way
for those others; so I hunted up the two boys
and said "they went out back one night to stone
the cat and fell down the well and got drowned."
Next I searched around and found old Aunt Patsy

Cooper and Aunt Betsy Hale where they were aground, and said "they went out back one night to visit the sick and fell down the well and got drowned." I was going to drown some of the others, but I gave up the idea, partly because I believed that if I kept that up it would arouse attention, . . . and partly because it was not a large well and would not hold any more anyway.

That was a long excursion—but it makes the point: that Mark didn't have much reverence for conventional story structure. Even his greatest book, which is perhaps also the greatest book written on this continent—*Huckleberry Finn*—is troublesome. One can scarcely find a criticism of the book which does not object, for instance, to the final episodes, in which Tom rejoins Huck and they go through that burlesque business of "freeing" the old Negro Jim— who is, it turns out, already free. But, as T. S. Eliot was, I think, the first to observe, the real structure of *Huck Finn* has nothing to do with the traditional form of the novel—with exposition, climax, and resolution. Its structure is like that of the great river itself—without beginning and without end. Its structural units, or "cages," are the episodes of which it is composed. Its momentum is that of the tension between the river's steady flow and the eccentric superimposed rhythms of Huck's flights from, and near recapture by, the restricting forces of routine and convention.

It is not a novel of escape; if it were, it would be Jim's novel, not Huck's. Huck is free at the start, and still free at the end. Looked at in this way, it is clear that *Huckleberry Finn* has as little need of a "conclusion" as has a skyscraper or a jazz performance. Questions of proportion and symmetry are as irrelevant to its structure as they are to the total effect of the New York skyline.

There is not room here for more than brief reference to the other "literary" items on our list: Whitman's *Leaves of Grass*, comic strips, and soap opera. Perhaps it is enough to remind you that *Leaves of Grass* has discomfited many a critic by its lack of symmetry and proportion, and that Whitman himself insisted: "I round and finish little, if anything; and could not, consistently with my scheme." As for the words of true poems, Whitman said in the "Song of the Answerer"—

They bring none to his or her terminus or to be
    content and full,
Whom they take they take into space to behold the
    birth of stars, to learn one of the meanings,
To launch off with absolute faith, to sweep through
    the ceaseless rings and never be quiet again.

Although this is not the place for a detailed analysis of Whitman's verse techniques, it is worth noting in passing how the rhythm of these lines rein-

forces their logical meaning. The basic rhythmical unit, throughout, is a three-beat phrase of which there are two in the first line (accents falling on *none, his,* and *term . . . be, tent,* and *full*), three in the second (*take, take,* and *space . . . hold, birth, stars . . . learn, one, mean*), and three in the third (*launch, ab, faith . . . sweep, cease, rings . . . nev. qui, gain*).

Superimposed upon the basic three-beat measure there is a flexible, non-metrical rhythm of colloquial phrasing. That rhythm is controlled in part by the visual effect of the arrangement in long lines, to each of which the reader tends to give equal duration, and in part by the punctuation within the lines. For example, the comma pause after the second three-beat measure in line two (after *stars*) tends, since the first line consisted of two such measures, to establish an expectation of rest which is upset by the line's continuing for another measure. Then, in the final line, the placement of the comma pause reverses the pattern, requiring a rest after the first measure and doubling up the remaining two.

It is the tension between the flexible, superimposed rhythm of the rhetorical patterns and the basic three-beat measure of the underlying framework which unites with the imagery and the logical meaning of the words to give the passage its restless, sweeping movement. It is this tension and other analogous aspects of the structure of *Leaves of Grass*

which give to the book that "vista" Whitman himself claimed for it.

If I may apply to it T. S. Eliot's idea about *Huckleberry Finn*, the structure of the *Leaves* is open at the end. Its key poem may well be the "Song of the Open Road," as D. H. Lawrence believed. "Toward no goal," Lawrence wrote. "Always the open road. Having no direction even. . . . This was Whitman. And the true rhythm of the American continent speaking out in him."

As for the comics and soap opera, they too—on their own frequently humdrum level—have devised structures which provide for no ultimate climax, which come to no end demanded by symmetry or proportion. In them both there is a shift in interest away from the "How does it come out?" of traditional storytelling to "How are things going?" In a typical installment of Harold Gray's *Little Orphan Annie*, the final panel shows Annie walking purposefully down a path with her dog, Sandy, saying: "But if we're goin', why horse around? It's a fine night for walkin' . . . C'mon, Sandy . . . Let's go . . ." (It doesn't even end with a period, or full stop, but with the conventional three dots or suspension points, to indicate incompletion.) So too, in the soap operas, *Portia Faces Life*, in one form or another, day after day, over and over again. And the operative word is the verb "faces." It is the process of facing that matters.

America Is Process

Here, I think, we are approaching the central quality which all the diverse items on our list have in common. That quality I would define as a concern with process rather than product—or, to re-use Mark Twain's words, a concern with the manner of handling experience or materials rather than with the experience or materials themselves. Emerson, a century ago, was fascinated by the way "becoming somewhat else is the perpetual game of nature." The universe, he said, "exists only in transit," and man is great "not in his goals but in his transitions."

This preoccupation with process is, of course, basic to modern science. "Matter" itself is no longer to be thought of as something fixed, but fluid and ever-changing. The modern sciences, as Veblen observed forty years ago, cluster about the "notion of process," the notion of "a sequence, or complex, of consecutive change." Similarly, modern economic theory has abandoned the "static equilibrium" analysis of the neo-classic economists, and in philosophy John Dewey's instrumentalism abandoned the classic philosophical interest in final causes for a scientific interest in the "mechanism of occurrences"—that is, process.

It is obvious, I think, that the American system of industrial mass production reflects this same focus of interest in its concern with production rather than

products. And it is the mass-production system, *not* machinery, which has been America's contribution to industry.

In that system there is an emphasis different from that characteristic of handicraft production or even of machine manufacture. In both of these there was an almost total disregard of the means of production. The aristocratic ideal inevitably relegated interest in the means exclusively to anonymous peasants and slaves; what mattered to those who controlled and administered production was, quite simply, the finished product. In a mass-production system, on the other hand, it is the process of production itself which becomes the center of interest, rather than the product.

If we are aware of this fact, we usually regard it as a misfortune. We hear a lot, for instance, of the notion that our system "dehumanizes" the worker, turning him into a machine and depriving him of the satisfactions of finishing anything, since he performs only some repetitive operation. It is true that the unit of work in mass production is not a product but an operation. But the development of the system, in contrast with Charlie Chaplin's wonderful but wild fantasy of the assembly line, has shown the intermediacy of the stage in which the worker is doomed to frustrating boredom. Merely repetitive work, in the logic of mass production, can and must be done by machine. It is unskilled work which is doomed by it, not the worker. More and more skilled

workers are needed to design products, analyze jobs, cut patterns, attend complicated machines, and coordinate the processes which comprise the productive system.

The skills required for these jobs are different, of course, from those required to make handmade boots or to carve stone ornament, but they are not in themselves less interesting or less human. Operating a crane in a steel mill, or a turret lathe, is an infinitely more varied and stimulating job than shaping boots day after day by hand. A recent study of a group of workers on an automobile assembly line makes it clear that many of the men object, for a variety of reasons, to those monotonous, repetitive jobs which (as we have already noted) should be—but in many cases are not yet—done by machine; but those who *like* such jobs like them because they enjoy the process. As one of them said: "Repeating the same thing you can catch up and keep ahead of yourself . . . you can get in the swing of it." The report of members of a team of British workers who visited twenty American steel foundries in 1949 includes this description of the technique of "snatching" a steel casting with a magnet, maneuvered by a gantry crane running on overhead rails:

In its operation, the crane approaches a pile of castings at high speed with the magnet hanging fairly near floor level. The crane comes to a stop somewhere short of the castings, while the mag-

net swings forward over the pile, is dropped on to it, current switched on, and the hoist begun, at the same moment as the crane starts on its return journey. [And then, in words which might equally be applied to a jazz musician, the report adds:] The whole operation requires timing of a high order, and the impression gained is that the crane drivers derive a good deal of satisfaction from the swinging rhythm of the process.

This fascination with process has possessed Americans ever since Oliver Evans in 1785 created the first wholly automatic factory: a flour mill in Delaware in which mechanical conveyors—belt conveyors, bucket conveyors, screw conveyors—are interlinked with machines in a continuous process of production. But even if there were no other visible sign of the national preoccupation with process, it would be enough to point out that it was an American who invented chewing gum (in 1869) and that it is the Americans who have spread it—in all senses of the verb—throughout the world. A non-consumable confection, its sole appeal is the process of chewing it.

The apprehensions which many people feel about a civilization absorbed with process—about its mobility and wastefulness as well as about the "dehumanizing" effects of its jobs—derive, I suppose, from old habit and the persistence of values and tastes which were indigenous to a very different

social and economic system. Whitman pointed out in *Democratic Vistas* ninety years ago that America was a stranger in her own house, that many of our social institutions, like our theories of literature and art, had been taken over almost without change from a culture which was not, as ours is, the product of political democracy and the machine. Those institutions and theories, and the values implicit in them, are still around, though some (like collegiate gothic, of both the architectural and intellectual variety) are less widely admired than formerly.

Change, or the process of consecutive occurrences, is, we tend to feel, a bewildering and confusing and lonely thing. All of us, in some moods, feel the "preference for the stable over the precarious and uncompleted" which, as John Dewey recognized, tempts philosophers to posit their absolutes. We talk fondly of the need for roots—as if man were a vegetable, not an animal with legs whose distinction it is that he can move and "get on with it." We would do well to make ourselves more familiar with the idea that the process of development is universal, that it is "the form and order of nature." As Lancelot Law Whyte has said, in *The Next Development in Man:*

> Man shares the special form of the universal formative process which is common to all organisms, and herein lies the root of his unity with the rest of organic nature. While life is main-

tained, the component processes in man never attain the relative isolation and static perfection of inorganic processes . . . The individual may seek, or believe that he seeks, independence, permanence, or perfection, but that is only through his failure to recognize and accept his actual situation.

As an "organic system" man cannot, of course, expect to achieve stability or permanent harmony, though he can create (and in the great arts of the past, has created) the illusion of them. What he can achieve is a continuing development in response to his environment. The factor which gives vitality to all the component processes in the individual and in society is "not permanence but development."

To say this is not to deny the past. It is simply to recognize that for a variety of reasons people living in America have, on the whole, been better able to relish process than those who have lived under the imposing shadow of the arts and institutions which Western man created in his tragic search for permanence and perfection—for a "closed system." They find it easy to understand what that very American philosopher William James meant when he told his sister that his house in Chocorua, New Hampshire, was "the most delightful house you ever saw; it has fourteen doors, all opening outwards." They are used to living in grid-patterned cities and towns whose streets, as Jean-Paul Sartre observed,

are not, like those of European cities, "closed at both ends." As Sartre says in his essay on New York, the long straight streets and avenues of a gridiron city do not permit the buildings to "cluster like sheep" and protect one against the sense of space. "They are not sober little walks closed in between houses, but national highways. The moment you set foot on one of them, you understand that it has to go on to Boston or Chicago."

So, too, the past of those who live in the United States, like their future, is open-ended. It does not, like the past of most other people, extend downward into the soil out of which their immediate community or neighborhood has grown. It extends laterally backward across the plains, the mountains, or the sea to somewhere else, just as their future may at any moment lead them down the open road, the endless-vistaed street.

Our history is the process of motion into and out of cities; of westering and the counter-process of return; of motion up and down the social ladder— a long, complex, and sometimes terrifyingly rapid sequence of consecutive change. And it is this sequence, and the attitudes and habits and forms which it has bred, to which the term "America" really refers.

"America" is not a synonym for the United States. It is not an artifact. It is not a fixed and immutable ideal toward which citizens of this nation strive. It has not order or proportion, but neither is it

chaos except as that is chaotic whose components no single mind can comprehend or control. America is process. And in so far as Americans have been "American"—as distinguished from being (as most of us, in at least some of our activities, have been) mere carriers of transplanted cultural traditions— the concern with process has been reflected in the work of their heads and hearts and hands.

The Curriculum
of Discovery*

* This essay is revised from an address given at the commencement exercises, Rhode Island School of Design, June 2, 1956, and subsequently published by the college in pamphlet form.

HERE IS A JOKE from a recent issue of a college magazine. A prospective employer says to a job applicant, "Yes, I'll give you a job. Sweep out the store." "But I'm a college graduate!" the young man protests. "Okay," comes the withering reply, "I'll show you how."

There it is: the distrust of non-technical, non-practical education. It is still around, even in these days of national concern about aid to higher education. It lurks in the background of much of the lip service paid to the "liberal arts" as opposed to "vocational" courses. And not without reason.

A century ago an almost impassable chasm existed between the interests and values of the everyday world of work and those of higher education as epitomized by the liberal arts. But there were increasing numbers of men of affairs and educators who saw, from their antipodal points of view, that the split was disastrous. On every hand there were demands that education must become more practical, meaning more immediately relevant to the concerns of an industrial society. Charles W. Eliot was about to re-orient Harvard's curriculum in ways

which were to have widespread effects throughout our educational system, introducing new subjects in the curriculum and loosening the old "classical" bonds. At about the same time separate institutions for advanced scientific and technical training, such as M.I.T. (where Eliot had taught before he went to Harvard) and the Rhode Island School of Design, were founded on the theory that no amount of juggling with the traditional curriculum would suffice for the training of men and women competent to deal with the highly specialized techniques and processes of modern civilization.

As a result of all this, the sum total of higher education became more closely related to the world of business and industry than it had been, but within education itself the split between "practical" and "cultural" studies remained. Indeed, in many instances these distinct aspects of learning became the province of separate institutions, as with the Sheffield Scientific School and Yale. Where both did manage to exist under the same roof, they were uneasy collaborators, full of mutual suspicion and distrust. In spite of appearances, the chasm between industry and culture was as wide and as deep as ever.

Looking back on it now, we can see that in a society which dissociates the technical and humane skills, both suffer. We know that in Europe and America, the practical world tended for more than a century to depend too exclusively upon technical skills, with the result that business and industry and

the spheres of life they dominated were in a measure dehumanized. What we less often recognize is that the world of culture, on the other hand, shunning the new environment of man's workaday life, turned in upon itself, marrying itself to its own past. And the more it did so, the more anemic and impotent it became.

If the symbol of one of these worlds became the "satanic mills," the symbol of the other became the mortuary grandeur of the museum. And in the field of education it was the liberal-arts curriculum which too often became a museum, as grand as it was inanimate.

In our lifetimes, events have made it impossible for the scholar and artist to maintain their isolation from the industrial and technical environment, or for the "practical" man to ignore the problem of values which are the province of liberal arts when they are alive and procreative. Much has been done in recent years to bridge the gap which had widened during the preceding century; but bridging a gap and closing it are not the same thing, and in that respect much remains to be done.

The Erudite Outsiders

When those trained in the liberal arts and humanities first began to turn their attention sympathetically to the problems and potentialities of modern industrial civilization, they were handicapped

by the fact that they were outsiders looking in. Their interest and their rapidly increasing knowledge tended to be theoretical. It was not founded upon what William James called "knowledge of acquaintance"—that is, knowledge derived from firsthand experience of a situation or a fact. What they proceeded to build up, therefore, in such fields of study as sociology, economics, and even in such fields as artistic and literary criticism, was "knowledge about" the dynamic areas of modern life, or erudition: the kind of knowledge that is derived not from firsthand experience but from reflection and abstract reasoning.

Both knowledge-of-acquaintance and knowledge-about are essential for the educated man or woman. Neither is in the long run adequate without the other. But knowledge of acquaintance—the empirical, practical kind—has at least this temporary advantage over the other: it can be put straight to work. Erudition, on the other hand, by itself, is often pragmatically useless, is mere words. In that simple fact lies the justification for that joke about the businessman's assuming that the college graduate wouldn't know how to cope with a broom.

The problem facing the educator is that though knowledge-of-acquaintance is not difficult to acquire, it is very difficult to teach. As Elton Mayo of the Harvard Business School pointed out some years ago, erudition can more easily be passed on to others than knowledge which depends upon trial and

error, example and imitation. And that is one reason why the academic profession in general prefers erudition to the other kind of knowledge.

But the educator's prejudice in favor of erudition has other and deeper roots. To a degree few of us would now willingly acknowledge, our preference relates back to the old snobbishness with which cultivated people looked down upon the merely practical problems of business and trade. Notice, for example, that almost the only area of liberal-arts education where knowledge-of-acquaintance as well as erudition is insisted upon is in the sciences, which are the newest part of the liberal arts curriculum. In physics, chemistry, psychology, and so on, laboratory work goes hand in hand (as it should) with the fruits of reflection and abstract reasoning. In the older parts of the curriculum—in history, literature, and the older social studies—only tentative and experimental moves have been made toward devising effective equivalents of laboratory work.

The result is that, in the liberal arts and humanities, our colleges are still a long way from providing that kind of education which young people in our industrial civilization require and deserve if we expect them to provide leadership for it. Anyone who doubts this would do well to look at the results of a survey on higher education published in *Fortune* several years ago. A representative sample of American parents was asked why they wanted their sons and daughters to go to college, and what they

wanted them to get out of it. The answer, both for sons and daughters, was overwhelmingly: preparation for a better job, or for a trade or profession; greater earning power. Only two per cent spoke of wanting their sons to get "culture, appreciation of the arts," and only four per cent wanted their daughters to get it.

There is a grim warning in this for those of us who think that it is to the liberal arts that men must look for that rounded development which may, under favorable circumstances, enable them to think logically and imaginatively, to understand their fellows and make themselves understood, to apply ideas to specific situations, and to make appropriate value judgments. It means that the pressures for getting on with the world's work still threaten to rob us of the time we need to consider the directions in which we want that work to take us. It is no wonder that, in a time when public opinion sets such high store by technical skill, the colleges find it so difficult to get financial support for work in humanities and the arts. We are in danger of forgetting that he who keeps his nose to the grindstone may get the immediate job done but may also grind away his nose, to spite his fate, if not his face.

Lest we become too despondent, however, there is another side to the picture. The leaders of industry and business—the practical men—are increasingly aware that technical skills without the humane skills to direct them are not adequate even for purely

practical and limited ends. Not long ago a large engineering corporation made a survey of its key executives' educational backgrounds. It found (as any good liberal-arts professor could have prophesied it would) that few of them came from technical schools; one was an apostate divinity student, one an ex-vaudeville man, and the majority came from liberal-arts colleges. Graduates of technical schools were invaluable in subordinate posts, carrying on the specialized aspects of the corporation's work, but they rarely rose above that level.

The Deadly Routine of Mere Skill

From both sides of the chasm, then, the need for closing the gap between knowledge-of-acquaintance and knowledge-about is recognized. But what have the educators done in the face of such evidence? Too often the technical and vocational schools have simply added to their curricula a few courses in literature or history. Similarly, the liberal-arts colleges too often have merely added a few practical courses (like "Writing for the Radio" or "Business English" or "Applied Psychology"). What it amounts to is that the vocational institution tells its students that in addition to the "useful" courses they came to school to get, they must also take some useless ones. And the liberal-arts colleges, panic-stricken at the rise of vocationalism and envious of the largesse which industry and government distrib-

ute to encourage practical and technical training, tell the job-conscious student that if he will just come and submit peaceably to culture, they will slip him a few useful courses on the side. The net effect, of course, in both instances, is that the gap between the technical and humane skills remains about as wide as before.

No society, least of all an industrial one, can master its enemies—or itself—if it depends for leadership upon men and women who are lopsidedly trained. I would wholeheartedly agree with my Columbia colleague, Jacques Barzun, that it is extremely dangerous to have the control of an industrial civilization rest in the hands of technical experts, or as he describes them, "a large, powerful, and complacent class of college-trained uneducated men."

Just as fearful, however, would be the prospect of depending for leadership upon members of a select, self-confident class, so stuffed with the kind of erudition which an enfeebled liberal-arts tradition often imparts that they had only contempt for the values (including the aesthetic and moral values) inherent in industrial civilization. Yet it is this contempt—a systematically supercilious contempt—which a good deal of so-called liberal-arts education still, in spite of its high intentions, tends to produce.

A great deal, I think, depends upon people who

have experienced a blend, or compound, of both kinds of training. It is good to get practical and technical training, to have opportunities to gain knowledge-of-acquaintance. It is good, also, to have opportunities to look through some of the doors which are opened by the liberal arts, because in so far as we avail ourselves of those opportunities, we will find that we are free. Free from the deadly routine of mere proficiency and skill; free from the threat of obsolescence which inevitably accompanies any technique in a civilization as mobile and changing as the one in which it is our destiny and our opportunity to live.

We hear a great deal about the need for more experts, more technically trained specialists: engineers, nuclear physicists, and so on. Only by training such specialists, it is said, can we preserve and defend our civilization against its enemies. Maybe so; but I doubt it. Nations or individuals who commit themselves to specialized techniques, no matter how advanced those techniques may be, lock themselves into rigid assumptions and expectations which some more adaptable and more imaginative nation or individual will inevitably upset. Techniques, whether in warfare or the arts or industry, are the ruts left by imaginative activity and disciplined thought en route to doing something. As long as that something is worth doing again, the ruts are worth following. But the capacity to follow them has little

to do with the capacity to determine when and for how long something is worth doing, or with the power to discover, among all the things that have never been done before, what is worth doing next.

Liberal Crafts and
Illiberal Arts*

* This essay is a revision of a keynote address given at the third annual Conference of American Craftsmen, June 20, 1959. Part of it was published in the October 1959 issue of *Industrial Design*.

IMPLICIT IN MUCH THAT WE SAY, and in many of the things we make and do, there seems to be the assumption that whatever is wrong or disappointing about the industrial society in which we live can be cured, or at least ameliorated, by reviving or adapting the values we inherit from a reputedly happier time when society was based upon agriculture and handicraft commerce. In the field of education this assumption underlies a good deal of the pleading for more attention to the liberal arts. In our discussions of the material products of our culture, it underlies our glorification of craftsmanship as opposed to mass production.

Science and technology, upon which industrial production rests, are commonly thought of as at best neutral agents (atomic energy is neither good nor bad in itself; it is what the politicians or generals or doctors do with it that matters). At worst they are thought to be anti-human (the assembly line), tending inevitably to dwarf our individuality and reduce us all to mechanical fragments in an irrational chaos. Either way, science and technology look pretty scary, and a society based upon them is obviously

in need of a good strong infusion of those time-tested values which the liberal arts and the handcrafts preserve and cultivate.

Much has been written in recent years about the role of education in preserving and fostering the heritage of the past, but less has been said about the contemporary interest in the crafts and in craftsmanship as a manifestation of a similar attitude toward the past. The concern with craftsmanship is obviously a significant feature of our time. Automobiles manufactured in plants which are the epitome of mass-production technology are advertised in terms which appeal to the buyer's admiration for the unique values of craftsmanship. The New York *Times* recently reported that a California company is doing a good business in little plaques to be attached to the dashboards of Plymouths and Pontiacs, which read: "Especially manufactured for . . ." with your name inserted. The term "artsy-crafty" may be a contemptuous epithet to fling at the non-functional and spuriously antique, but we speak of "the arts and crafts" with increasing respect.

Those who call themselves craftsmen seem to fall into two groups. There are the one-of-a-kind makers, who by and large avoid machines except those which, like the hand loom or the potter's wheel, are sufficiently ancient to have acquired non-industrial associations. And there are the craftsmen who design and make objects which may serve as models for production-line manufacture. Both groups

appear to share the wish, or determination, to contribute to our industrial civilization certain values
(or, more specifically, certain qualities of form and
color and texture) which were evolved in pre-industrial society and whose loss—or neglect—would
diminish our pleasures or, worse still, deprive us of
perceptions which can enrich our lives. One group
seeks to do this by reviving or carrying on the actual
handcrafts, with all their qualities of uniqueness—
making things and perpetuating processes in direct
(and often successful) competition with the things
and processes of industrial technology. The other
group, in the spirit of missionaries to the industrial
heathen, carries the gospel into the factories themselves and seeks to reshape the products of industri-
alism in the image of the crafts.

The assumption that we can learn from the past
how to correct what is wrong in industrial society is,
generally speaking, an article of faith among all sorts
and conditions of men. One encounters it everywhere
from the *Reader's Digest* to the *Partisan Review*,
from editorials in the Chicago *Tribune* to the Harvard report on *General Education in a Free Society*.
At a recent symposium on "The New View of Man"
to which notable scholars in many fields contributed,
a distinguished liberal-arts professor produced a
paragraph which can serve as a characteristic sample of the spontaneous overflow of anti-technological
emotion. He was talking about the split between the
artist and society. And, like everyone else, he traced

91

that split to the industrial revolution, which during
the past century and a half has "mechanized our
lives and our outlook." Perhaps out of deference to
some of his faculty colleagues he conceded that science and technology had brought "immense gains"
to mankind. But with that concession out of the way,
he went on to say that we'd have to admit "that the
old way of life [the pre-industrial way] was natural,
and that life in the modern megalopolis is unnatural."

> A man and his family are no longer, even in the
> country, a self-sufficient community, living close
> to a stable tradition and the processes of nature,
> but are mobile, isolated, rootless atoms, depend-
> ent upon a multitude of external agencies. Un-
> less he makes a determined effort, an effort
> that invites the label of eccentricity, modern
> man loses the use of his hands and his feet and
> his senses, not to mention the time and capacity
> for reflection.

In contrast with all this, he said, art "starts from the
natural activity of man's natural faculties . . . its
values are not the values of a mechanized, acquisitive society."

I have quoted at such length because the rheto-
ric of this passage fascinates me. The tune is so
familiar we could all whistle it, once we have heard
the opening measures. It is full of haunting phrases
which remind us of one another, like the songs of our

childhood: "self-sufficient community," "stable tradition," and "close to nature" (the slight variation on this last phrase, "close to the processes of nature," won't throw anyone off the tune), and, in a sort of simple counterpoint with these nostalgic bits, we hear "mobile, isolated, rootless," "loses the use of his hands and feet," and "no time for reflection." (I missed "frenetic hurry" and "robot" in this last sequence—but one can't have everything.)

Before we examine the paragraph further, I should, however, make clear that it is not typical of the essay from which I have extracted it. The essay deals thoughtfully with the role of literature and of the writer in our society, not with technology and science, and the author is a professor of literature, not a student of society or the history of technics. But that is precisely why this paragraph is useful to us here: it is a completely unself-conscious compendium of the clichés which leap to our tongues when we feel sentimental about the good old days of literature, art, and craftsmanship. As such, it is worth a look, to see if the assumptions underlying the clichés have any coherent relevance to the state of affairs in which we find ourselves.

Natural Arts and Unnatural Sciences

What does it mean to say that man's life in pre-industrial society was "natural," while the life of man today is not? Is it not "natural" for man to make

tools, and to power those tools with machines, and to use those tools to remake his environment? What is "unnatural" about being mobile? Were we not born with legs and endowed by nature with minds capable of conceiving of the wheel and a motor to drive it? Is mobility on wheels less "natural" than mobility on legs, or only less brutish and more "human"? And what is unnatural about a rootless atom? Could there be anything more unnatural than an atom *with* roots? Are a man and his family who have television, a car, and a telephone really more "isolated" than those who herded sheep in Palestine two thousand years ago, or those who lived in eighteenth-century English country houses? Are stable traditions more natural than unstable ones? And are the processes of nature, to which we like to think of being close, really stable or, as Werner Heisenberg's "uncertainty principle" in modern physics suggests, at best relatively so? And isn't it curious that a society which has deprived all but the eccentric of the use of their feet and hands and senses, regularly cracks the four-minute mile, buys fishing rods and skis in unprecedented quantities, operates turret lathes and typewriters with dextrous grace, and has learned to respond creatively to sensory stimuli which, without the microscopes and X rays and other resources technology and science have put at our disposal, man would never have seen or felt or heard?

In short, are not all of these deprecatory comparisons of the "natural" life of the old days with

the "unnatural" life of our own society either meaningless or—worse—a sentimental refuge from thinking about the challenge which our society really offers us? For there is a challenge involved, as there
always has been and always will be. Life attends to
that.

The paragraph ends by saying that since art
starts from "the natural activity of man's natural
faculties" its values have nothing in common with
those of our mechanized, acquisitive society. I hope
it is clear that in so far as this stereotyped conclusion
rests upon the notion that there is something unnatural about contemporary society, it is highly suspect. But there are two more points to be made.

The first is that, if the writer means what he
says, he is sounding the death knell of art. For he has
said that the values of art have no relevance to the
values of a "mechanized, acquisitive society" and
he has said that we are living in just such a society.
Society is us; if society's values are not those of art,
the values of art are not ours, and we can and will
dispense with it. That, in cold logic, is what the
paragraph says, but we would agree, I think, that it
is not what the author meant.

What did he mean? Or, to bring the problem
to our own doors, what do we mean when we say
things like that? We mean, I suppose, very little more
than that there are times when it seems that too
many people don't care enough about the things we
design or write or paint, or about those books or

paintings or other artistic achievements which have given joy and perceptive understanding to many people in the past and which still have the capacity to give such joy and understanding. Some of us are so anxious to coddle our pride in our lonely sensibility that when thirty million people watch *Hamlet* on TV some evening, we quickly find ways to belittle the fact. We point out that it was, after all, a capsule *Hamlet*, reduced to an hour and a half—as if that proved that the thirty million wouldn't have watched for two and a half or three hours if the producers had been able to afford or get the time. Of course it may be true that if the whole play, uncut, had been televised on a three-hour program, only fifteen or twenty million would have watched; but it is also true that there might have been thirty-five million. We can't be sure. What we can be sure of is that no comparable fraction of the total population of the English-speaking world ever deliberately exposed themselves to *Hamlet* in any "natural" state of society before the industrial revolution. It may be a pity that an even larger fraction of the possible TV audience watched other shows that night, instead. But even here I think we should be careful not to be too sure. Maybe what they were watching was worth watching. The chances are good, if Shakespeare's career means anything, that the profoundest and most enduring creative work of our time will be done —as his was—for a popular medium of entertainment. If it is, there is not much chance of its being seen,

or appreciated, or encouraged by those of us who mourn the sorry fate of art in our mechanized, "unnatural" times. It often seems to me that if art needs any defending, it needs defending from those of us who call ourselves its friends; against its enemies, I am sure, it is quite capable of defending itself.

We do no one any good by indulging in sentimental stereotypes about the inferiority of our society to the societies of the past. We simply confuse ourselves, discourage the creative artists (if they take us seriously), and lead the general public to conclude (quite justifiably) that if art is, as we seem to find it comforting to think, something which only people like us can enjoy, we're welcome to it.

This brings me to the second and final point about the paragraph from which I have quoted. Toward the end of it, the author uses two terms to characterize our society. He calls it mechanized and acquisitive. At the beginning he had talked as if it was the mechanization introduced by science and technology which made industrial society at odds with the artist. Now, suddenly, a new element—acquisitiveness—is introduced, and introduced in such a way that it is made to seem like just another name for mechanization, as if a society which is mechanized is *ipso facto* acquisitive.

Those who remember Veblen's classic distinction between the acquisitive motives and the motives of production and service will have already detected the irony of this verbal juggling. For mechanization

and acquisitiveness have nothing in common, and the values of a society based upon science and technology are in the profoundest sense at odds with those of an acquisitive society.

Is It Natural to Be Human?

We come face to face, at this point, with the basic challenge our society presents to us. Is it, in fact, a society whose values are primarily shaped by science and technology? To the extent that it is so, it is something new under the sun, and makes unprecedented demands upon those who do its work, direct its dynamic forces, and give artistic expression to its aspirations and doubts. If it is merely an acquisitive society, a business society rather than an industrial one, and if it is motivated primarily by the desire for power and pecuniary gain, there is nothing new about it. In that case it may well be true that the moral problems confronting the modern individual are essentially the same as those which have confronted individuals in the past, and that the insights and perceptions contained in the literature and art which have come down to us from the ancient East, and through the long tradition of Western culture, provide us with the most direct and powerful illumination of life's meaning and its potentialities.

The challenge society presents to us is the challenge to look about us, with minds and senses un-

clouded by stereotyped responses, and to think and speak and act in unhackneyed response to what we see. If we can accept this challenge, we may discover that the society we live in really is, as we frequently say it is but seldom believe it is, founded upon and shaped by technology and science. To the extent that it *is* so founded, it is a society which puts a premium upon adaptability, mobility, and a willingness to forego the security of fixed status and the certainty of dogmatic absolutes. For technology and science always and everywhere make for change. They are not mere collections of machines and test tubes, but processes by which we change our environment and thereby change ourselves. They are therefore the ineluctable enemies of all the static, traditional features of society as men knew it in the past—the enemies of all varieties of vested interest, of all the habitual and ceremonial aspects of institutions, of all fixed systems of dogma, whether the dogma be religious, political, or aesthetic.

It would be surprising indeed if, in such a society, the arts of the past, expressing very different values, should not in some important respects seem less relevant than they once seemed. And it would be still more surprising if the reputations of some artists, who once seemed of the first importance, should not dwindle while those of others (such as El Greco and Blake) should be enhanced.

Similarly, it would be inconceivable that the artists and craftsmen of our own time, whether they

are working in traditional modes or in the new media which have been provided by technology itself, should not express in their creations those values which our society demands. For what society wants, society gets.

A society based upon science and technology wants artists and craftsmen and workers whose values are relevant to the type of interdependence which science and technology require of mankind. As Walt Whitman knew a century ago, the "American" world (whose boundaries, as I have suggested, are not by any means limited to those of the United States) demands a new individuality—an individuality freed from ceremonial homage to dead certainties and imaginatively responsive to the challenge of "a revolutionary and future-founding age."

Fifty years ago, Simon Patten, a pioneer of economics in America, delivered a series of lectures on *The New Basis of Civilization,* one of which concludes with a relevant passage. Science and technology, Patten said, had already, by 1905, "fundamentally altered" the elemental relations between man and nature which had formerly existed. To say that the methods which have made men physically independent of the local climate and the local food supply, which have given him control over nature in so many respects, are artificial or "unnatural," was, Patten said, to underrate the powers of technology and science "by implying that they are constantly

opposed by fundamental natural forces which in the end must again triumph." The triumph of man's scientific and technical intelligence over the materials of nature was to Patten as "natural" as any other step in the evolution of life on earth.

> Each gain upon nature [he wrote] adds to the quantity of goods to be consumed by society and lessens the labor necessary to produce them. In one form the surplus is stored in individuals as surplus energy; in another it is in the goods produced by this energy. . . . The surplus is not conserved as a permanent fund, but exists and grows only as it is perpetually transformed from goods to energy and from energy back to goods. . . . It relieves the present from the menace of a deficit which our forefathers constantly faced and feared. As a concept of our social thinking it differentiates the new from the old and helps to drive away the mists that blur clear thinking.

Reading these words written in 1905, those of us who remember the great depression of the thirties, and the horrors of two world wars brought on in part by nations of men who feared "the menace of a deficit," may conclude that Patten was naïvely optimistic about the future of a society based upon man's scientific and technical mastery of nature's materials. Such a conclusion is unwarranted, unless we can demonstrate that it was the new bases of

society which caused the depression and the wars, and this would be hard to demonstrate. Patten was by no means naïvely optimistic about the immediate future, and the wars would not have surprised him. The concept of surplus energy would, he said, "help to drive away the mists that blur clear thinking" about society and its possibilities, but as he promptly went on to say, "states of mind are hard to change, and in truth those we so long ago adopted seem to find ever fresh justification in the evils which remain to afflict men long after their inciting causes have disappeared; in the old wounds of humanity it is easy to see new proofs of accustomed beliefs."

> We know [he said] that the military state is gradually being displaced by the industrial state, and yet there never was a time when the power and efficiency of armies was as great as now. . . . And so it is with the evils more directly associated with the industrial world. The poverty, misery, exploitation, oppression of the poor; the greed, indifference, and power of the rich, are glaring truths even while the basis of a new economic order becomes more and more plain. In the age of transition the old thought and the new world abide side by side. But if the foundations of our civilization have been changed, the altering status of men will take clearer aspect in each new age, and the old thought, while apparently verifying the old

premises anew, will gradually disappear—not because it is argued away, but because men's sentiments are changed by new activity and an accumulating store of fresh experiences.

As a teacher, I know Patten was correct in saying that the old thought, the old states of mind, cannot be argued away. I know also that in great measure the educational system in which I play a part is still dominated by the values and states of mind of a time when men were under the domination of nature, and when it was therefore essential to train their hands to overcome, and their minds to transcend, the savagery of land and water. It is an education which, as Patten knew, "teaches that beauty is in medieval craftsmanship, and ugliness in the machine-made object," and which turns the student toward the abstractions of logic and the consolations of historical study in all fields.

I know also, that the great task of education, and the great challenge to artists and craftsmen, is to arouse man to the domination of his new, man-made environment—the urban world of the industrial megalopolis—"by stimulating eye and ear until he sees and hears fresh inducements to activity" and by making him acquainted with the unimagined possibilities of a world which, if strange, is strange only because we have not yet quite dared to believe that to be human in ways which control nature is quite natural to human beings.

Farewell, Architecture!*

SPECIALIZED ART
IN A VERNACULAR CULTURE

* This essay incorporates material from two earlier papers. Some of the material was originally written to be read before the Architecture Society of the Rhode Island School of Design, on November 3, 1958, and was published by the society in a pamphlet entitled *Whatever Became of Architecture?* Most of the rest is revised from the summation address at the First Pacific Rim Conference, sponsored by the California Council of the American Institute of Architects, held in Honolulu, Hawaii, October 8–14, 1959, and published in the *Architectural Record*, April 1960.

ARCHITECTURE SEEMS TO BE a flourishing art. New buildings are going up in all our cities. A number of architects are well-known figures, and most members of the profession appear to be prospering. But a diminishing fraction of our architecture is the work of architects. Most buildings are designed (if that isn't too flattering a term) by builders, contractors, engineers, or industrial designers. Even those which architects claim to have designed are frequently in large part the work of such specialists as the structural engineers, heating and ventilating engineers, acoustical engineers, interior designers, and the public relations and marketing experts with whom architects form partnerships or whom they employ.

What first called my attention sharply to the architect's diminishing role in architecture was some statements I came upon in the annual of the Society of Industrial Designers, *U. S. Industrial Design 1951*. In the section on "Commercial Interiors and Exteriors" it is casually asserted, without the least tone of surprise or triumph, that "in recent years the members of the Society of Industrial Designers have be-

come increasingly active in certain fields that once were considered the exclusive province of the architect." In these activities they are serving not only their established clients but "many corporations which have not yet retained industrial designers for any other type of assignment."

The matter-of-fact tone in which this information is conveyed is, from the point of view of a layman interested in architecture, astonishing. But even more astonishing is the fact that, so far as I am able to discover, no architect and no architectural publication was astonished by it.

Why is it that industrial designers are increasingly being called upon to take over jobs formerly done by architects, even for clients who do not hire industrial designers to do what they are set up to do? Why have industrial designers, not architects, been asked to design not only ships, trains, and airplanes, but also theaters, service stations, retail shops, department stores, and corporate administration buildings? How does it happen that it was Raymond Loewy who got the job of designing Filene's largest branch store, or Walter Dorwin Teague who got the job of designing the first joint project ever undertaken by two major stores—the co-ordinated suburban stores of S. S. Pierce and R. H. Stearns in Chestnut Hill outside Boston, for which Teague designed and executed the entire complex, including plot-treatment, buildings, interiors, and fixtures?

The design annual's answer to these questions

is simply that none of these structures is primarily an architectural project. "Architecture here," it tells us, "is merely a technique of creating or enclosing a functional machine, and in each case the machine must be made efficient and attractive by exactly the same methods employed to make a manufactured product successful on the market." To the design of anything from a department store to a city, the industrial designer, we are told, applies exactly the same processes he is accustomed to apply in designing a refrigerator or an office machine. "It is precisely because [he] follows this unconventional procedure," according to the annual, "that he is now finding so many opportunities to do so."

Two things strike me as of special interest to architects in this argument. One is the implication that by taking over the job of "creating or enclosing" functionally organized space the industrial designer is not really doing anything that is of interest to architects. An architect's blood would, I should think, curdle at the word *merely* in the assertion that—so far as department stores and office buildings are concerned—the technique of creating or enclosing functional space is merely incidental. For if architecture is not that, what on earth is it?

The other thing worth noting is that there is not the slightest indication that the spokesman for the industrial designers wants to claim credit for them as architects. On the contrary, he is at pains to say explicitly that the industrial designer "does

not claim to be an architectural specialist." (Notice
that word *specialist.*) What he is proudly and clearly
asserting is that industrial designers have a distinct
and "unconventional" procedure, a "proved technique," with no resemblance to the procedures and
techniques of architecture. If they are called upon to
do jobs which people called architects used to do,
that is just common sense, because the jobs are not
those with which an "architectural specialist" would
be concerned.

What, then, is the "proved" technique, the "unconventional" procedure, employed by the industrial
designer? The answer, according to the annual, is
that the technique is one of applying certain processes of analysis and synthesis. And this technique is
then outlined in a paragraph which implies as much
about the limitations of contemporary architects as
it tells us directly about how an industrial designer
works.

The paragraph opens with this sentence, in
which that blood-curdling word *merely* crops up
again: "Building design—which is merely a process
of deciding how a given space shall be enclosed—is
the last thing the industrial designer thinks of when
he is asked to design a building." Without the slightest overtone of malice or aggressiveness, quite matter-of-factly, this sentence says that the sort of thing
architects specialize in is entirely an external and
superficial matter, of no immediate concern to an
industrial designer faced with the job of designing

a building. "Building design," in the context of the industrial designer's thought, is something you don't bother about until you have done the really important job, which is "to design a building."

The "unconventional procedure" which the industrial designer follows in designing a building such as a department store is then outlined thus:

> He first wants to know exactly what is to be done and accomplished in the space to be enclosed. . . . Here there is so much area to be allotted to each type of merchandise, and each must have certain special facilities and settings for storage, display, and selling; these departments have a logical relationship to each other, and while they become in effect a series of specialty shops, the transition from one to another must be easy, natural, comfortable. There are certain logical points at which customers will enter the premises; there is a desirable sequence in which the facilities of the store should be presented to the customer's attention; the customer's comfort and convenience must be considered at every point . . . a thousand details of operation must be provided for efficiently and unobtrusively.

Only after he has considered all these and innumerable other requirements, has discussed them with management, reconciled them with each other, and organized them in a satisfactory scheme, does

the industrial designer "determine the structure that will enclose the whole." And even then, the annual tells us, he must be influenced by many "practical considerations," as opposed, one assumes, to aesthetic ones, such as the necessity for adequate identification (signs), for displays designed to attract the passer-by, for convenient and sheltered entrances and exits, for easy access to parking places, and so on. With the net result that his exterior design, when he gets to it, "grows naturally out of a balance of these requirements."

The Ideal Architect

What strikes me about this description of the industrial designer's "unconventional procedure" is its similarity to what was formerly thought to be the architect's function. Five centuries ago Leone Battista Alberti, the Florentine architect and architectural theorist, said that any common workman could "run up" a building "that is immediately necessary for any particular purpose, and about which there is no doubt of what sort it should be, or of the ability of the owner to afford it," but that "to raise an Edifice which is compleat in every part, and to consider and provide beforehand everything necessary for such a work" is the business of an architect.

"Him I call an Architect," Alberti said, "who . . . is able . . . to devise, and, with execution, to compleat all those works which . . . can . . . be

adapted to the uses of mankind . . ." That (in Leoni's eighteenth-century translation) is the skeleton of the fifteenth-century humanist's definition of an architect. The essential elements of this definition are, I suppose, two: that it is the architect's job to devise and to complete the structure, and that the structures must be humanly useful.

I repeat, however, that this is only the skeleton of Alberti's definition. There are, in fact, five places where I have cut away from the basic structure of Alberti's thought those phrases by which he qualifies and extends its meaning. The full quotation reads as follows:

> Him I call an Architect, who, by a sure and wonderful Art and Method, is able, both with thought and invention, to devise, and, with execution, to compleat all those Works, which, by means of the movement of great Weights, and the conjunction and amassment of Bodies, can with the greatest Beauty, be adapted to the uses of Mankind: and to be able to do this, he must have a thorough insight into the noblest and most curious Sciences.

I quoted the grammatical skeleton, the basic framework of his conception, first by itself, without the subordinate qualifications and extensions, to emphasize the degree to which Alberti's conception of the architect subordinates the idea of Beauty to that

of usefulness, and to call attention to the tremendous importance he attaches to a knowledge of the techniques of construction and planning. Notice that the architect's ability to "devise and compleat" his works is limited by three separate qualifications. First, he is able to do it only if he has the mastery of "a sure and wonderful" combination of art (by which Alberti means technique) and method. Even then he is not *able* unless he employs both thought and invention. (That word *invention,* of course, does not mean what we would call creative imagination; it is a technical term, in common use during the Renaissance to mean the disposition of the various conventional elements of a composition in new and appropriate arrangements.) Having interrupted himself twice to specify prerequisites to the architect's ability to "devise and compleat" his useful works, Alberti seems, for the moment, satisfied. But no sooner has he got to the end of his thought than he remembers still another reservation he wants to make. Art and method, thought and invention, are not, after all, enough to enable the architect to do his job. He must also have "a thorough insight into the noblest and most curious sciences." If he has all these things, he is able to build structures which can be adapted "with the greatest beauty" to the uses of mankind.

I do not want to underplay the significance Alberti attaches to "Beauty," about which he says a

good deal in Book VI and Book IX of his treatise. "Beauty and ornament" (he likes to refer to them in tandem) are the sources of the "pleasure and delight" we take in looking at buildings. Beauty he defines as the harmony or congruity of all the parts of a structure; ornament he defines as something "added or fastened on" so that the unsightly parts of a structure will give less offense and the handsome parts will be even lovelier. (He therefore calls ornament a kind of "auxiliary brightness and improvement to Beauty.") In one place he even says that the architect's having satisfied necessity by his structure "is a very small matter," and that even if he has also achieved "conveniency" his building will give no pleasure if people are shocked by its "deformity." But when he returns to the subject later, he is careful to restore the balance. It should always be clear, he insists, that the architect has "consulted necessity and convenience in the first place."

First and foremost the architect is, in Alberti's phrase, the "Inventor of all Conveniences." Mankind, he tells us, is obligated to the architect not only for safe and pleasant shelters, but for having "contrived" many other things "of the highest use and convenience," such as sweat baths; aqueducts; tunnels; ships and vehicles; bridges; and engines of war. More victories in war, he says, have been won by the "art and skill" of the architects than by the conduct or fortune of the generals.

Versatility versus Specialization

The Renaissance flavor of all this, its undismayed recognition of the need for versatility, may well seem naïve to those of us who have been constantly reminded that ours is an age of specialization. We know (or at least we think we know) that a man who knows enough to build a bridge can't possibly know enough besides to design a church, let alone a sweat bath. Perhaps that is so; but it may be useful to entertain some doubts about it.

For myself, I wonder if our abject acceptance of compartmentalization and specialization is not in part the result of an understandable but disproportionate reverence for science. The sciences are, of course, highly specialized—so much so that it is almost impossible in an academic community to get the physicists and biologists and chemists and experimental psychologists to approve any joint offering, or even to endorse any course in the history of science. Their reluctance is soundly based in that it is quite literally impossible for any one person to know enough to be both a chemist and an experimental psychologist. The rise of such nominally overlapping sciences as bio-physics and bio-chemistry, far from being a sign of a unification of the sciences, is rather a sign of still greater specialization. A biologist or a physicist, I am told, could no more swap

laboratories with a bio-physicist than a geologist could swap places with a botanist.

It is to specialization of this sort that we are indebted for much knowledge (or, more accurately, for vast quantities of relatively reliable data) about our world and ourselves. Architects know, as well as the rest of us, that the structures they design owe much to the data provided by highly specialized sciences. And by a peculiar distortion of logic they, like all of us, seem to conclude that, if specialization can produce such valuable data, it can do anything.

But of course it can't. It can produce data on the strength of materials, but it can't use the data. It can produce data on the psychological effects of texture and color, but it has no way of putting such data to use. As J. Robert Oppenheimer has bravely said, scientific knowledge, "by the very techniques, powers, and facts of its acquisition [which is to say, by its highly specialized procedures], precludes other knowledge." He points out that in a physics laboratory, for example, the kind of arrangement that is suitable for doing an experiment to find out *where* an atom is, precludes the possibility of acquiring knowledge about the rate at which it is moving. Not only does learning where a given atom is make it impossible to learn its velocity; it also, Oppenheimer tells us, "makes it logically contradictory to assume that the other quantity (i.e., velocity) has a value."

Scientific data can be acquired, in short, only by a system of rigid specialization. It is no wonder,

therefore, that specialization has come to be honored and respected and—most important of all—enjoyed. The kind of knowledge which science can acquire—knowledge which is reliable to a relatively high degree—is, as Oppenheimer justly says, incredibly precious. And to the scientist the specialized procedure with which he acquires this knowledge—the process of acquiring it—understandably becomes an end in itself. "It is just the technique and the wonder of one's own ability to do it" that is for Oppenheimer "part of the value of it."

This delight in process is a characteristic feature of our American world. But scientific processes are not the only ones in which man may find delight, and neither the architect nor the physician nor the teacher nor the corporation executive nor the politician (nor the scientist, for that matter) need conclude that the only respectable or fruitful processes are those which, like the processes of science, are highly specialized. It is at least possible that, at this moment in history, the processes of synthesis and generalization may be even more fruitful than those of specialization.

By suggesting this possibility I do not wish to imply that I have any use for the notion, which even some very eminent scientists have flirted with, that there should be a moratorium on science. There cannot ever be too great a quantity of relatively reliable data available to mankind, though I am well aware

that there may be too much for a given individual to cope with.

It does seem to me, however, that the individual's difficulty in coping with the flood of new data which has poured out of the scientists' laboratories is compounded by a mistaken sense that he has no right to the fruits of specialized techniques unless he has mastered the techniques by which they were produced. We tell one another, in dozens of ways, that this is so. In an agony of self-depreciation we tell ourselves that we should be ashamed if we drive cars whose inner functioning we do not understand, or if we listen to music emitted by a device whose electronic complexities are beyond us. In part this sense of guilt is the result of the scientists' own insistence that the popularization (or making generally available) of the results of their highly specialized techniques is naughty and disreputable, and in part it is simply the result of a vestigial puritanism which makes us feel guilty about having anything which we didn't earn by the sweat of our bodies or minds. As if life itself were not a gift.

There are, of course, very good reasons why all of us, including architects, should be aware of the distinction between firsthand and secondhand knowledge. But there are also very good reasons why we should not try to require of ourselves a firsthand knowledge of all the data upon which we form our judgments and decisions. Which is simply another way of saying that we must all be (as in fact we

all are) generalists as well as specialists. There are also good reasons why, in these days, some of us should specialize in being generalists. Which is another way of saying we need architects, in Alberti's sense of the term, as well as poets and philosophers.

The Heart as Nucleus

Thanks, in part at least, to the idea of specialization, the procedures which to Alberti seemed to distinguish an architect from a common workman now seem, to the industrial designers, to distinguish them from architects. If the industrial designers are correct, it is no wonder that they are being asked to undertake jobs which architects would formerly have been expected to do. Nor is it surprising that Buckminster Fuller, who has designed some of the most creative and elegant structures of this century, should emphatically insist that he is not an architect but "a research department for architecture." One is reminded of the "thorough insight into the noblest and most curious sciences" which Alberti's architect had to have.

I have discussed these matters with friends who are architects, but they do not seem to be alarmed by having lost to industrial designers a few commissions for stores, chains of service stations, and airliners. They have plenty to do anyway, and if they have any uneasiness about what is happening they cover it by slightly disdainful references to the

industrial designers' penchant for publicity. With all respect for the professional honor of the architects I happen to know, I have never noticed that architects in general are unduly hampered by professional ethics in calling attention to themselves and their talents. One has heard of Frank Lloyd Wright and Mies van der Rohe.

But one has also heard that Mies's roofs leak, and that in the kitchen of Wright's masterpiece, the Imperial Hotel, things were so designed that there was no way to get at and clean up the bug-heaven of food and grease which accumulated behind the ill-placed stoves. Small matters, these, when set against the visual delight which Mies and Wright have created by "building design." But if I were footing the bill for a new apartment house or hotel, not to say a gas station or airliner, I would probably turn, however regretfully, to a designer who thought *first* about the "comfort and convenience" of the people who would use it, and about providing "efficiently and unobtrusively" for the thousand and one details of the operations (including living) which would be carried out in it.

Nor would I assume, in making my choice, that I was thereby running a great risk of getting a structure which, though efficient and convenient, was likely to be deformed and unsightly. I remember Thoreau's observation that whatever architectural beauty he saw about him had "gradually grown from within outward, out of the necessities and character

of the indweller . . . without ever a thought for the appearance"—and when I remember it, I do not think it is perverse or romantic nonsense. It reminds me in turn of Horatio Greenough's admonition to American architects over a century ago: "Instead of forcing the functions of every sort of building into one general form, adopting an outward shape for the sake of the eye or of association," let us, he said, "begin from the heart as a nucleus, and work outward." I take the word *heart,* in this passage, in both its senses.

Ballerinas in Polo Coats

To the extent that the architect combines in his own person the builder and the engineer as well as the artist, to the extent, in other words, that he exemplifies Alberti's ideal and has avoided the illusion that the specialization essential to science is also desirable in the arts—to that extent he will be directly responsive to the life about him. But the architect as specialist, as designer pure and simple, seems to be primarily responsive not to life but to architecture.

The idea that artists may be more responsive to art than to life was first suggested to me by a remark made by a very great teacher when I was in graduate school. The teacher was Mark Van Doren, lecturing on epic poetry. He had the great teacher's gift of saying things parenthetically, in the midst of some-

thing else he was saying, which did not interrupt the main thread of his discourse but which later grew and developed in fascinating profusion—as if the enclosing parenthesis formed a sort of pot in which the planted idea could germinate while the lecture went on, and in which you could take it away afterward, if you wanted to, and watch it grow.

What he said parenthetically on this occasion was, if I remember correctly: "Of course poetry is not inspired by life, but by other poetry. It is not the girl you are in love with who inspires you to write a sonnet, but some sonnet you have read about some other girl." I remember being horrified by the remark because I had just written a sonnet about a girl and wanted very much to believe it was a direct response to her charms. Some years later, however, I came upon that sonnet and ruefully discovered no trace of the flesh and blood girl in it though there were some painfully evident traces of one of the limper sonnets of John Keats.

To a considerable extent what Mark Van Doren said is true not only of poetry but of all the arts. Each of us, of course, instinctively seeks to arrange the elements of his environment in satisfying patterns of color, sound, texture, and so on, and a human being who was cut off from acquaintance with traditions of art would promptly set about improvising patterns and forms of his own. But in a society where we are surrounded by paintings, music, poems, and architecture it is impossible to respond

to the unadorned reality about us with senses un-affected (or should I say untrained) by our prede-cessor's selectively ordered reflections of it. It is prob-ably not a landscape, but a painting of a landscape, which drives the incipient painter to canvas and brush. So too the incipient architect is probably in-spired less by the physical, social, and cultural reali-ties of his environment than by the work of his fellow architects, living and dead.

Van Doren's comment raises, of course, the question of how, if art is initially inspired by art rather than by life, art ever got started. Obviously someone must at some point have produced a paint-ing in direct response to a human figure or a natural landscape, because at some point there can have been no other paintings to prompt him. There must have been a first house, a first temple, a first pyramid, designed (or improvised, if you prefer—though the terms are more nearly synonymous than we usually admit) as a direct response to physical factors and to such basic social needs as those for shelter, for wor-ship, or for the assurance of immortality. The forms which have been developed and refined, echoed and re-echoed in our various traditions of design, obvi-ously had their origins in primordial responses to physical and social realities, unhelped and unhin-dered by earlier formal solutions.

Once a formal solution has been found, of course, it tends to be repeated; and the better the solution is, the more it will affect subsequent build-

ings. In architecture, as in the other arts, it is with forms developed over a long period by many craftsmen that the creative artist works. It is these traditional forms which provide him with the vehicle for his perceptions. They serve him as the conventions of ballet serve the dancer, and become in effect the conventional costume he puts on while dancing his own dance. A ballerina wearing the standard frilled *tutu* and moving in a traditional *pas de deus* is a good deal freer to express her unique vision than one wearing a polo coat.

I am sure there must be an architectural equivalent to what Robert Frost said about the exigencies of traditional verse forms. As Frost put it, writing poetry without rhyme or meter is like playing tennis with the net down.

Frost's remark is especially useful in our context because it permits us to ask whether there are not other nets than traditional English rhyme and meter which may put zest into the game of poetry. And of course, a number of poets, including such diverse figures as Walt Whitman, greatest of American poets, and the Japanese haiku writers from Matsuo Bashō to Masaoka Shiki, played the game with nets very unlike the traditional net of English verse and very unlike each other's.

There are those who would argue that it is one thing for a Japanese poet, who belongs after all to a different culture, to use a net unlike the one we are used to, but quite another thing for Whitman (and

his successors) to do so. Whitman seems to them, as it were, a traitor to his class, willfully seeking a flatulent originality. The literary argument roughly parallels the architectural one which has been employed in Henry Hope Reed, Jr.'s, recent book denouncing modern architecture in all its manifestations, on the ground that it has merely seceded from tradition in a fruitless effort to be original. The author passionately recommends instead a new courthouse for San Francisco in what is called "the high classical manner," with "rusticated arched entrances, marked keystones, gold lanterns, and statues in profusion," all designed by a man identified as (and I quote) "an interested amateur who resides in Berkeley, across the bay."

In a sense the argument is sound. If we assume that the American world we live in is the same world whose "life" originally inspired the forms which were refined and developed by the great artists of the past, there is indeed no excuse for an urgent search for new or significant forms. The artist will employ the forms indigenous to his culture, as Milton and Wordsworth employed the sonnet form, not fretting at their "narrow gloom" but rejoicing in the knowledge that he has at his command vehicles relevant to the experience of his fellow men, in which he can express his own personal vision of life's abiding charm, or wonder, or horror (for all three, I am afraid, abide). As long as there is a basic continuity in the culture, the traditional forms retain a valid

relation to the vital forces in contemporary life. Modifications will, of course, be necessary as time brings gradual change. But there is no danger that artistic conservatism will resist them effectively. Society has plenty of built-in devices to induce even the most recalcitrant architect to adapt his work in some measure to contemporary reality—one of the most effective, the client's bank roll.

But what if the world we live in is not a mere evolutionary modification of the culture which dominated the Western world a thousand years ago? What if the world we still sometimes think we are living in has been so transfigured by unprecedented influences that it is in effect a new ethnical epoch? What if technology and science really have made fundamental changes in man's relation to the natural world about him, to his fellow men, and to God?

There have been times during the past century or so when people talked as if technology and science *had* produced such fundamental changes. But it is characteristic of the persistence of our mental and emotional habits that people in general have not acted as if they believed it, and have generally refused to listen if anyone spoke bluntly about the consequences. At the turn of the century, for example, the American engineer and bridge builder, George S. Morison, wrote a moving and impressive book arguing that the discovery of ways to manufacture power had initiated changes which during the next couple of centuries would be more far-reaching

than any brought about by earlier epochal advances such as the use of fire, the domestication of animals, or the invention of written alphabets. Writing in 1898, Morison foresaw that the new technology would bring almost inconceivable changes not only in material ways but in man's social and intellectual life. Let me quote a brief passage:

> The manufacture of power . . . has separated power from the mind which must manage it; it calls for intelligent design and direction of the multitude of works which it has rendered possible; it has equipped our generation with tools for study and investigation as well as for mechanical work. The new epoch will alter the relations between the professions, business, and trades; it will readjust the duties of government and the relations of one government to another; it will change our system of education.
>
> . . . The new epoch differs from all preceding epochs, in that while they represented successive periods of progress, different races existed simultaneously in every period of advancement, whereas the new epoch must from its very nature soon become universal . . . It brings all races together, and must in time remove all differences in capacity.

This quoted passage deals in generalizations; but Morison's book is specific. Referring to architecture, for example, he notes that the manufacture

of power "has made the demands of the new epoch so different from those of the old that nearly everything which has to be used must be built anew." In the new epoch, he said, "architecture, which as a fine art would consign itself to the museum, and which sometimes, following the rapid changes of fashion, seems to differ from millinery chiefly in the want of a beautiful object on which to place its novelties, will find its highest development in correct construction."

One would have thought that in the days when the Bauhaus influence was in its ascendancy, architectural theorists would have rediscovered Morison's book, and perhaps even given some attention to the house he designed and built in Peterboro, New Hampshire. But they did not, and I suspect that the reason is that he was too blunt in his insistence that the new epoch is really new. We all talk wistfully at times about "a new heaven and a new earth," and to generations of men "the new world" has seemed, at moments at least, to be a social and cultural possibility as well as a geographical reality. But the new is unfamiliar, and unfamiliarity as well as familiarity breeds contempt. When we move into our new glass box we are likely to take grandmother's rocker and somebody else's grandfather's cobbler's bench along with us.

I suppose that our basic dislike and distrust of the new epoch and the emergent forms appropriate to it is the result of two facts: first, that as Morison

foresaw, it has opened as an era of destruction. He understood that the new epoch would "from its very nature destroy many of the conditions which give most interest to the history of the past, and many of the traditions which people hold most dear." Looking back from our moment in time, we can see that he was right in prophesying that there would be, for perhaps a century or more, "great destruction of old buildings, old boundaries, and old monuments, and furthermore of customs and ideas, systems of thought and methods of education." And destruction is sad—so sad that, like death, it sometimes appears to us to be tragic.

The destruction has come, and will continue, not, Morison said, because the things which are destroyed are in themselves bad, but "because however good and useful they may have been in the past, they are not adapted to fulfill the requirements of the new epoch." The danger is that the destructive changes will come so fast that the new developments, appropriate to the new world, do not come fast enough to fill the gap between them. And of course such developments (in architecture, education, or whatever) will not come fast enough if, each time we are frightened by some destructive change, we decide that change itself is bad and that we must therefore renounce all attempts at new solutions and go back, as the phrase is, to "the high classical manner," or the theology of Aquinas, or the politics of Aristotle, or whatever the "unchanging verity" in our neck of the woods may be.

The Wellsprings of Design

It is my conviction that the society we live in marks—as Morison said it did—a really new epoch, but that it is shaped not by technology and science alone but by a unique combination of forces, a compound of scientific technology and the spirit of democracy. Some years ago—more than a decade—I tried to suggest that these twin forces had been revolutionizing man's conception of his relations to nature, his fellow man, and his gods, for more than a century, and that the elements of the emergent environment produced by these twin forces were for many years shaped not by our artists but by untutored citizens working without any "artistic" pretensions. It is the patterns and forms these people evolved which the artists of our time must arrange (and have begun to arrange) in patterns and forms satisfactorily expressing the values and attitudes appropriate to the new epoch.

It was my contention that the early, unschooled attempts to create satisfying patterns out of these novel elements in our environment constituted a new kind of folk art. The folk arts we are familiar with are the product of groups cut off from the main stream of contemporary life, and they are the surviving remnants of traditional forms and patterns. These new "folk arts" are, on the contrary, the product of people directly involved with the dynamic forces of contemporary life, and their forms and patterns have

no precedent, since the environmental elements to which they give shape are quite literally something new.

In order to distinguish them from the more familiar folk arts, I labeled these the vernacular arts—meaning by that the empirical attempts of ordinary people to shape the elements of their everyday environment in a democratic, technological age. Specifically, I meant the books, buildings, and artifacts of all sorts whose forms have been shaped as a direct response to the new elements which democracy and technology have introduced into our environment within the past hundred and fifty years.

The buildings produced in such a vernacular tradition (as, for example, the early balloon-frame houses of the American Midwest) were often ugly. So it is easy for the admirers of the "high classical" manner in courthouses to dismiss them as "mere inventions in the construction industry" and to accuse those of us who are interested in them of writing the kind of architectural discussion which would consider Venetian architecture solely in terms of pile-driving. But this misses the point.

The point about the balloon-frame houses which came out of Chicago in the 1830's and spread all across America in the following decades, is that their builders empirically discovered a form which took full advantage of machine-made lumber and machine-made nails and machine transportation (three elements of the technological environment which tra-

ditional architecture had no use for), and a form, furthermore, which also incorporated the elements of economy, speed of construction, mobility, flexibility, and universal availability fostered by the spirit of democracy. And, finally, the point is that out of this anonymous, unrefined form, later architects evolved structures which, by any valid standards, are architecture of a very high order indeed, however unrelated they may be to the more massive and rigid architecture of hand-hewn beams and hand-hewn stone, incorporating the aristocratic and hierarchical values of order and stability.

We could illustrate the role of the vernacular in evolving new forms, appropriate to the new environment, by reference to other examples, including the steel frame and the concrete shell. But the point would be the same: that in a time of rapid and future-founding change, the architect who ignores the vernacular, with its unself-conscious and uninhibited response to the elements of a new environment, and who submits himself too devoutly to the inspiration of past architecture (his own, or that of others) runs a grave risk of losing fruitful contact with the life about him.

The risk is compounded, I think, in our time by the degree to which criticism of the arts is replacing the arts themselves as the source of artistic inspiration. I know that in the literary arts this is so, and I have the impression that just as there is a good deal of poetry which owes more to the critics than to

other poetry (let alone to life), so there is a good deal of architecture these days which owes more to what the writers in architectural magazines say than it does to the aesthetic realities. It would be a pity, I think, if we were to have a plague of architects who are less excited by architecture than by writers who are excited about architecture.

But if architects should, as Mark Van Doren's comment implied, properly take their inspiration from architecture, it seems important in these rapidly changing times that they include under that head not only the masterpieces of the past but, more especially, the humble vernacular which is springing up around them in direct response to the new elements which democracy and technology are continuously introducing into the lives of people everywhere. Architectural criticism generally admires the work of those whose work is cognate with the achievements of the great artists of the present and the past. But great artists never imitate their equals; they plagiarize from their inferiors.

If architects submit to the influence of the critics they will be hounded into the shadow of some imperious, though dead, perfection. But the perfection embodied in the great architecture of the past, as in the great poetry and great painting, is the culmination of a growth which began far back in the inexpert gropings of ordinary mortals. The forms which reached their loveliest and most moving expression in the Gothic cathedrals of the Middle Ages were

evolved not from those of classical temples but from those of common barns and markets, just as Beethoven's symphonies were an elaboration of formal elements originating in folk music, and just as Shakespeare's plays were the combination of a long development in the popular theater. We tend to forget that Shakespeare did not write *King Lear* because he was steeped in Aeschylus and Sophocles, but because he found in the crude forms evolved by generations of inferior predecessors a vehicle, relevant to his time, which he could adapt and refine so that it fitly conveyed a vision of life which his genius made relevant to all times.

Vernacular forms, whose elements are the materials and processes of technology and the attitudes and interests of democracy, will continue to be improvised wherever technology and democracy make themselves felt among the peoples of the earth. They will, of course, be modified in each region by physical and social actualities and by the local cultural heritage which goes deeply into the quality of what we build. But they will share the quality of immediate responsiveness to the driving energies of the new epoch. They will be crude, unrefined, and—if you will—ugly, more often than not. But they are the most life-giving of all the wellsprings of design, and if the architect indeed vanishes from the contemporary scene it will be because he mistook them for less.

What Is "American" in Architecture and Design?*

NOTES TOWARD
AN AESTHETIC OF PROCESS

* This essay is a revised and expanded version of an article published originally in *Art in America*, Fall 1958.

ALL OF US AT TIMES need to confirm the continuity of our culture with that of the past, in order to reassure ourselves in the midst of bewildering flux and change. The author of the so-called "uncertainty principle" in modern physics, Nobel prize-winner Werner Heisenberg, has himself felt such a need, and recently went to some length to "prove" that he owes his eminence in atomic physics to an early reading of Plato's *Timaeus* and a sound training in the Greek natural philosophers.

We may ask what is "American" in architecture and design because we want to establish their continuity with buildings and objects of the past. And if this is our motive in asking the question we will, of course, be most interested in those buildings and objects whose structure and aesthetic effect are clearly related to, and thus comparable with, those of their predecessors in the Western tradition. We will concern ourselves, that is, with architecture in its textbook sense, as a fine art which has developed continuously, with local and national variants, throughout the Western world.

If we approach the question in this way, taking "architecture" to mean churches, government buildings, and palaces (for princes or merchants), and taking "design" to include what the nineteenth century lumped as "Industrial Art" (manufactured objects to which one could apply "arts and crafts" decoration, such as pottery, textiles, bijouterie, and the printed page), we will probably conclude that the "American" quality is catholicity. We can find in the United States an imitation of almost any architectural style or decorative mannerism which ever existed in any other nation. And when we have done so, all we shall have demonstrated is what we already knew: that Americans came from everywhere, and brought with them the traditions—architectural and decorative as well as social and religious—of which they were the heirs. We shall have learned what is English or Spanish or German about our architecture and our design, and therefore how they relate to the Western tradition; but we shall know as little as ever about their "American" quality, if such there be.

There is, for example, nothing "American" about New York City's Cathedral of St. John the Divine, except perhaps the fact that it is unfinished. It is an important and lovely fact of our cultural history and of the history of architecture in this country, but it tells us more about what is not "American" than about what is, just as a Coca-Cola bottle made in

France tells us more about what is "American" than about what is French.

The question can be asked, however, not in hopes of establishing ties to the past but in hopes of discovering those elements of creative energy and vitality which can evolve forms and structures appropriate to a world of flux and change—the "American" world—even at the risk of devaluing or destroying much that we have cherished and loved in the past. If this is our motive, we must look at those structures and objects which were not thought of as "Architecture" or "Industrial Art" by those who designed or paid for them. We must look, in other words, at those structures and objects which have been unselfconsciously evolved from the new materials, and for the unprecedented psychological and social uses present in the "American" environment.

The Vitality of the Vernacular

If we go at the question in this way, we will discover, I think, that the "American" quality is the product of a vernacular which has flourished in the United States but is by no means confined to it, which has deep roots in Western Europe, and which is rapidly establishing itself wherever modern technology and democracy are working together to recast our consciousness of our relations to one another, to external nature, and to our Gods.

I am again using the term *vernacular* as a de-

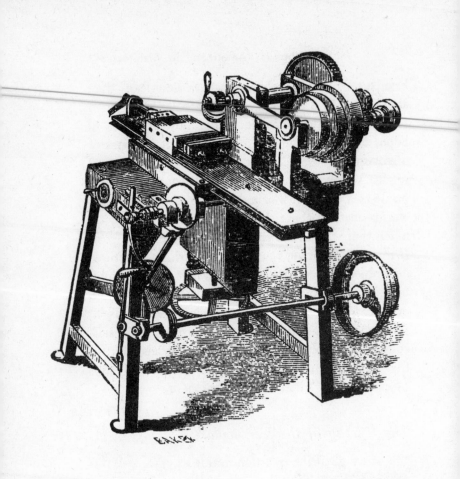

Above, Robertson's Milling Machine, Patented 1852 (from a wood
engraving in an advertisement in David Bigelow, *History of
Prominent Mercantile and Manufacturing Firms in the United
States,* Boston, 1857); *upper right,* A Brainerd Universal Milling
Machine of 1894 (from a wood engraving in *Illustrated Price
List* of the Fairbanks Co., 1894); and, *lower right,* the Cincinnati
Milling Machine Company's Universal Milling Machine of 1943
(from the *American Machinist,* May 27, 1943).

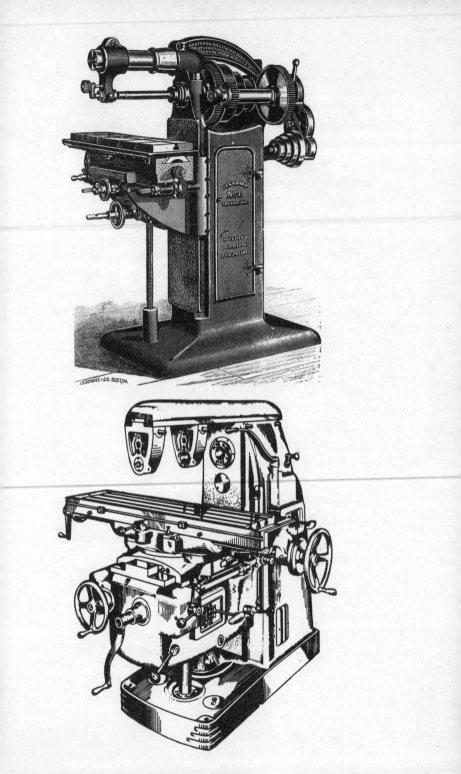

scriptive label for the patterns and forms which people have devised, usually anonymously, in attempting to give satisfying order to the unprecedented elements which democracy and technology have jointly introduced into the human environment during the past hundred and fifty years or so.

Actually there are two ways in which people can order the elements of a new environment. One is to cramp them into patterns or forms which were originally devised to order other and quite different elements of another and quite different environment. Hence the mid-nineteenth-century blank verse "epics" about backwoodsmen in Kentucky; hence the flying buttresses of Raymond Hood's Chicago Tribune Tower; hence "symphonic" jazz and amphora-shaped cigarette lighters. The forms or patterns in such instances will often have a symmetry and finish which give genuine (if nostalgic) pleasure, but only at the cost of considerable distortion of the elements which have been worried into them. It would be interesting to consider, for example, how we warped the development of a system of higher education appropriate to an "American" world by corseting it in pseudo-medieval cloisters and pseudo-Renaissance palaces.

The other way is to shuffle and rearrange the unfamiliar elements until some appropriate design is empirically discovered. The vernacular patterns or forms so devised will often be ungainly, crude, or awkward in contrast with those evolved and refined

over the centuries to order the elements of the pre-democratic, pre-industrial world, but they will at least bear a vital relation to the new environment of whose elements they are composed. More importantly, they will contain within themselves the potentiality of refinement and—God willing—of transfiguration by the hand of genius.

As an example of the characteristic evolution of vernacular form, we may take the development of a machine tool such as the milling machine. Three stages in its design are illustrated. The earliest machine shown in the series was made forty years after Eli Whitney created his first practical machine tool of this type, but it is still a gawky four-legged object which has not yet discovered the so-called "knee and column" form appropriate to its functions, in which both of the later machines are made. Bearing in mind that each stage in the development of this machine represents an advance in the magnitude and complexity of the operations it is designed to perform, even a non-mechanic will be able to observe the increasing simplicity and refinement of the over-all design.

If we turn from mechanics to building we may perhaps more easily see the way in which vernacular forms and patterns can become expressive elements in creative design. In the past thirty years many structural elements which were developed in vernacular building have become characteristic features of contemporary architecture. One has only to look

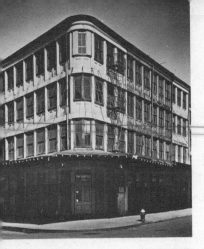

Left, Cast Iron Building designed and built by James Bogardus, 1848, on northwest corner of Washington and Murray streets, New York (photograph courtesy Gottscho-Schleisner); *below left,* The Hotel del Coronado, on San Diego Bay, California, 1889 (wood engraving from promotional pamphlet, *Coronado Beach,* Oakland, 1890); *below,* Abandoned Tobacco Factory in Louisville, Kentucky (photograph, 1943, courtesy of Reynolds Metal Co., which bought the building that year for conversion to aircraft-parts manufacture).

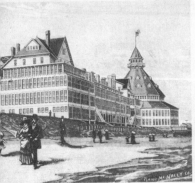

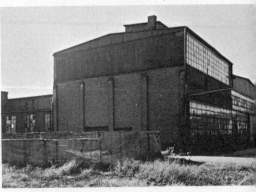

at the accompanying pictures of a century-old iron loft building, the glass-enclosed verandahs of a seaside hotel of the eighteen eighties, and an abandoned tobacco factory to be aware of the vernacular roots of important elements in the architectural design of such buildings as Albert Kahn's tank arsenal, the Farm Security Administration's utility building for a California migrant camp, and Raymond Hood's magnificent McGraw-Hill building—done after he had learned to dispense with the Gothic trappings of the Tribune Tower.

146

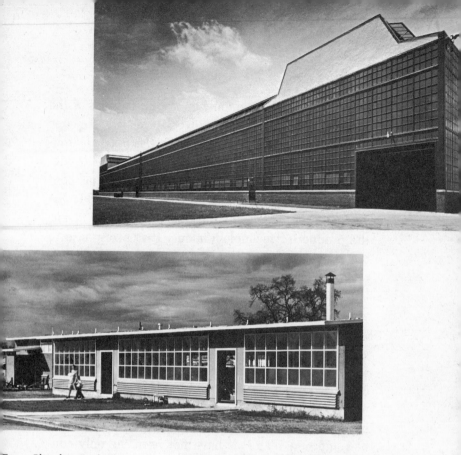

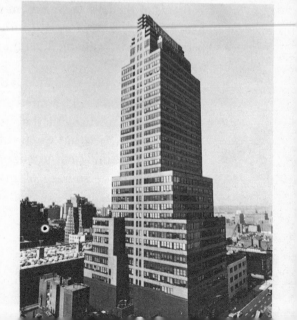

Top, Chrysler Tank Arsenal, designed by Albert Kahn, 1940 (Hedrich-Blessing Studio, courtesy of *Architectural Forum*); *above,* Utilities Building, FSA Camp, Woodville, California (photograph courtesy Library of Congress); *right,* The McGraw-Hill Building, West Forty-second Street, New York, designed by Raymond Hood, 1931 (photograph courtesy McGraw-Hill Studio).

Thus far we have touched upon examples of the vernacular which were evolved primarily to cope with or exploit those elements of the new environment which were introduced by technology—by developments in the machining of metal, in frame construction, and in the manufacture of glass. But the vernacular as I have tried to define it is by no means the product of technology alone. It is a response to the simultaneous impact of technology and democracy. Watt's first practical steam engine and the Declaration of Independence became operative in the same year, we should remember. Technology by itself can become the servant of a tyrant, as has been amply proved in Hitler's Germany and Stalin's Russia and, on a smaller scale, in some communities closer to home. But it is the peculiar blend of technology with democracy which produces vernacular as opposed to merely technological forms. New technics and new materials have not been the only constituents of the new environment for which men have had to discover appropriate forms. There have also been new amalgams of thought, of emotion, and of attitude.

If, for a moment, I may use the term "American" in its conventional and limited sense, as referring to whatever has to do with the United States, it is a very American fact that we are chiefly indebted to a European for calling our attention to the anonymous and "undignified" sources of many of the creative elements in contemporary architecture and design. It

was the Swiss scholar Siegfried Giedion, who, in the Norton lectures at Harvard in 1939, first showed many of us that such utilitarian structures as the balloon-frame houses of early Chicago, and such utilitarian objects as nineteenth-century water pails and railway seats, were often more prophetic of the essential spirit and creative force of our contemporary arts than the buildings and objects which have been acclaimed for their "artistic" quality.

By now it is clear that many of the constituents of contemporary design which at first struck us as alien and strange evolved from our vernacular. The molded plywood which seemed so startling when it appeared in chairs exhibited at the Museum of Modern Art in the late thirties and early forties was the conventional material for seats in American ferryboats in the 1870's. The spring-steel cantilever principle, which attracted world-wide attention when Mies van der Rohe used it in a chair he designed at the Bauhaus, had been standard in the seats of American reapers and mowers and other farm machines since the 1850's. Built-in furniture, the "storage wall," and movable partitions to create flexible interior space, all three were employed in an ingenious amateur house plan worked out in the 1860's by Harriet Beecher Stowe's sister, Catherine Beecher, a pioneer in the field now known as home economics. The provision of storage facilities in interchangeable units, which can be rearranged or added to, as changing needs and circumstances require, had a long

history in office equipment, kitchen cabinets, and sectional furniture before it was recognized as an appropriate element in creative design.

What is important about such instances, from the point of view of this article, is that so many of them reflect a concern with process, especially as it is manifest in motion and change; for it is this concern, as I have said, which seems to me to be central to that "American" quality which we are trying to define.

The Syntax of Momentum

Wherever we look in the field of the vernacular we will discover such designs. Let us look, for example, at a column of text from the first guidebook published for travelers on the transcontinental railroad, reproduced at right. No one, I suppose, would select such a page for inclusion in an exhibit of graphic arts; but if we examine it attentively we will discover many elements of typography and layout which tell us more about the dynamics of our civilization than any page we are likely to find included in the "Fifty Best Books of the Year" or any similar exhibit.

The general structure of the book from which it is taken (the *Great Trans-Continental Tourist's Guide . . . over the Union Pacific Railroad, Central Pacific Railroad . . .* , New York, 1870) is dictated, of course, by the westward journey. The main line

schools and churches are in a flourishing condition. The United States Branch Mint of Nevada is located at this place. The newspaper interest is represented by the Carson *Appeal*, a daily paper, which has long been established here.

Carson City is situated in the center of the best farming land on Carson river, and the best in this part of the State. Carson is connected by stage with Genoa, Markleville and Silver Mountain. A narrow-gauge railroad has been built from Carson to Virginia City, which will be pushed forward to a connection with the Central Pacific at an early day.

GENOA CITY,

Fourteen miles southwest from Carson, is a thriving town of about 500 inhabitants, situated in a fine section of farming country on the Carson river, on the stage road to

MARKLEVILLE,

A mining town, in the State of California, on the eastern slope of the Sierras, containing about 600 inhabitants.

SILVER MOUNTAIN,

Another mining town, 14 miles from Silver Mountain, containing about 400 inhabitants. The country abounds in silver mines around these towns.

Leaving the mines and Carson City, we once more return to Reno and resume our journey west. Near by Reno the hills are loftier, nearer the river, and covered with pine forests, and as we enter the canyon we seem to have entered a cooler, pleasanter, and more invigorating atmosphere. The aroma of the spruce and pine is pleasant when compared with that of the alkaline plains. It is related of an Eastern lumberman, from "away down in Maine," who had been very sour and taciturn during the trip across the plains, refusing to be sociable with any of his fellow travelers, that when he entered within the shades of the forest, he straightened himself up in the cars for a moment, looked around, and exclaiming, "Thank God, I smell pitch once more," sank back in his seat and wept for joy.

Among these hills, with the river rolling along on our right, we pass along merrily, the dry, barren desert, forgotten in the new scenes opening to our view, until we reach

VERDI,

A station 11 miles west from Reno. Elevation, 4,915 feet. On, up the river, with its foaming current, now on our left, first on one side, then on the other, runs this beautiful stream, until we lose sight of it altogether. The road crosses and re-crosses it on fine Howe truss bridges, running as straight as the course of the mountains will permit. The mountains tower up on either hand, in places, sloping and covered with timber from base to summit, in others, precipitous, and covered with masses of black, broken rock. 'Tis a rough country, the canyon of the Truckee, possessing many grand and imposing features. Occasional strips of meadow land are seen, close to the river's edge, but too small and rocky to be of use, only as grazing land. Now, we cross the dividing line, and shout

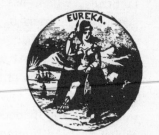

as we enter California, a few miles east of

BOCA,

A station, 16 miles west of Verdi. Elevation, 5,560 feet. The lumber interest is well represented here, huge piles of ties, boards and timber lining the roadside. The river seems to be the means of transportation for the saw logs, immense numbers of them being scattered up and down the stream, with here and

Facsimile of page 154 in the *Great Trans-Continental Tourist's Guide*, New York, 1870, the first guidebook published for passengers on the recently completed transcontinental railroad.

of narrative and description follows the moving train past towns, settlements, and natural features along the route, with digressive loops to include sidetracks and feeder lines—both stagecoaches and railroads. To help the reader keep track of where he is, and to make it easy to find the portions of the text dealing with particular localities or topics, the author—or typesetter—broke the type columns into sections, with subheads in capital letters. Early in the book these subheads are merely phrases which serve the familiar function of titles for sections dealing with such matters as THE FAR WEST, ROLLING STOCK, and LAND GRANT. But at the point where the actual journey by train begins, something happens to these subheads, typographically and syntactically, which has a good deal to do with the jazz-like sensation of momentum which the book produces. The change occurs near the end of the "chapter" of the text which is headed OMAHA. The general description of this town, which was the starting point for the trip on the new transcontinental railroad, is subdivided into various sections, each of which deals with some important aspect of the town. The last of these is headed OMAHA BARRACKS. Typographically it appears to be a section consisting of three paragraphs, followed by another section dealing with SUMMIT LANDING (A FLAG STATION); but that's not what really happens.

Paragraph three begins as if it were going to be, like its two predecessors, about the barracks. The

first sentence reads: "At present there is no chaplain."
But that is the only sentence about the barracks. The
next one, in spite of a conjunction which looks as if
it tied what follows tightly to the idea that there
was no chaplain at the barracks, gets us on board
the train and on our way:

> But we must take our leave of Omaha, as
> the whistle is sounding its warning signal
> to step into the cars and commence our
> journey over the plains to the far west.
> We pass along through the suburbs of the
> town for about four miles, when we arrive
> at
>
> ### SUMMIT LANDING
> ### (A FLAG STATION.)
>
> at an altitude of 1142 feet. We are leaving
> the busy hum . . .

What has happened here is that the typography
(like the syntax) has been overridden by the impe-
tus of the narrative. And from this point on, with
only occasional relapses into conventional treatment,
the subheads are not permitted to halt or slow the
westward momentum.

The designer of the layout—whether this was
the author or the typesetter—obviously does not
know, however, quite how to cope with this new
form which he has contrived—or which his material
has forced upon him. Sometimes he puts a period

at the end of the subhead, even though the words in it are grammatically a part of what follows; at other times he uses a comma.

Eleven miles further we arrive at

COLTON.

A new station six miles east of

SIDNEY,

Nebraska Territory. Company F, of the
ninth infantry is stationed here. . . .

Sometimes he uses a small letter, sometimes an un-called-for capital letter, to begin the new typo-graphical section; at other times he both indents and capitalizes the first word, even though there is no grammatical break whatever.

At first the subheads which are incorporated into this run-on pattern are the names of towns or settlements through which the train passes. After a while, however, the pattern becomes habitual and is extended to all sorts of topics and subtopics. And by the time we cross the boundary into California—in that part of the text reproduced here—an illus-tration, the seal of the state, is incorporated into the momentum of the narrative syntax. Crude as it is, this pattern of picture-text continuity, contrived al-most seventy years ago, is more "advanced" than anything we are likely to find in this week's slickest picture magazine. The anonymous designer who

stumbled upon it was no William Morris, either in his respect for craftsmanship or in his mistrust of the world which technology and democracy were collaborating to create. One may doubt that his knowledge of Greek philosophy and science went much beyond the Archimedean exclamation in the California seal, but the "American" world whose values and attitudes he shared, and for some of whose elements he improvised a suitable pattern, was one to which a world-view like that of mid-twentieth-century physics would not seem alien. It was a world which seems, in retrospect, to have been at least subconsciously aware that, as Werner Heisenberg said in a recent lecture on *Quantum Theory and the Roots of Atomic Science*, energy is the substance from which all things are made; that "energy is in fact that which moves; it may be called the primary cause of all change."

The Aesthetics of Process

In an earlier essay I have tried to show that the quality shared by all those things which are recognized, here and abroad, as distinctively "American"—from skyscrapers to jazz to chewing gum—is an awareness of, if not a delight in, process: that universal "process of development" which, as Lancelot Law Whyte has said, man shares with all organic nature, and which forever debars him from achieving the perfection and eternal harmony of

155

which the great arts of Western Europe have for centuries created the illusion. In the hierarchical civilizations of the past, where systems of status kept people as well as values pretty much in their places, men were insulated against an awareness of process to an extent which is no longer possible. In an environment dominated by technology and democracy, a world of social and physical mobility and rapid change, we cannot escape it. And our awareness of process is inevitably reflected in the vernacular, just as our occasional dread of it is witnessed by our continuing commitment to the cultivated forms inherited from a world in which permanence and perfection seemed, at least, to be realities.

It is the ideas, emotions, and attitudes generated by this conscious or unconscious awareness of process which account, I think, for a basic difference between the aesthetic effects of vernacular forms and those of the cultivated Western tradition. Inevitably, the forms appropriate to our contemporary world lack the balanced symmetry, the stability, and the elaborate formality to which we are accustomed in the architecture and design of the past. They tend, instead, to be resilient, adaptable, simple, and unceremonious. Serenity gives way to tension. Instead of an aesthetic of the arrangement of mass, we have an aesthetic of the transformation of energy. Only in some such terms as these, it seems to me, can we describe the so-called "American" quality which we detect in our architecture and design.

What Is "American" in Architecture?

It is not possible in a brief essay to do more than suggest the implications of such an approach to the question asked in our title. Obviously it restricts our attention to a limited field of structures and objects, and diverts it from some of the most charming and interesting things which have been produced in this country. But it has the merit, I think, of converting a question which can easily become a mere excuse for a naïvely nationalist antiquarianism, or an equally naïve internationalism, into one which may help us discover the aesthetic resources of an "open-ended" civilization, of an "American" environment which reaches far beyond the borders of the United States. It also has the modest merit of requiring us to look with fresh eyes at things around us—not just the things in the decorators' shops and museums, but the humbler things which, because the people who made them took them, as we do, for granted, are often spontaneously expressive of those elements in our environment which do not fall naturally into traditional forms and patterns.

One way to emphasize the point I am trying to make is to contrast a product of the vernacular with a masterpiece of the cultivated tradition. Books on the architecture of bridges do not, so far as I know, refer to structures such as the bridge built in 1882 across the Canyon Diablo in Arizona, on what is now the Santa Fe Railroad. Seen in contrast with the majestic Pont du Gard, one of the most

perfect examples of Roman masonry construction, which rises 155 feet above the river Gard near the French city of Nîmes, this spider-web truss of iron, carrying heavy locomotives and cars 222 feet above the bottom of the canyon, dramatically illustrates the utterly different aesthetic effects produced in response not only to new technics and materials but also to new attitudes and values. The two structures, embodying fundamentally different conceptions of time, of space, of motion, and of man's relation to external nature, make essentially different demands upon our attention.

If we can put aside, for the time being, all question of which structure is the more beautiful, there will be no difficulty in recognizing which of the two is embodied in a scheme of forms that is capable of becoming a vehicle for an architecture expressive of the American environment.

In the triumphant composure of its daring triple arcades the aqueduct calmly declares that by its completion, almost two thousand years ago now, its builders had accomplished, once and for all, a tremendous task. Hewn stone lies on hewn stone or thrusts diagonally downward against hewn stone, each held immovably in place by its own dead weight. The railroad bridge, by contrast, is entirely preoccupied with what it is doing. Its trusses and girders are a web of members in tension and members in compression, arranged in supple, asymmetrical equilibrium. The stones of the aqueduct rest there,

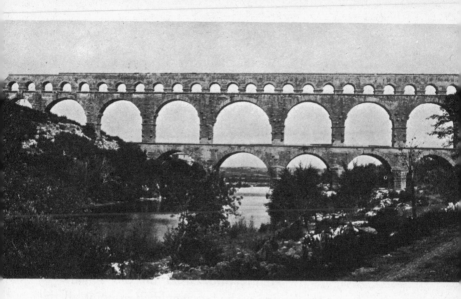

The photograph of the Pont du Gard, near Nîmes, France, is reproduced from Charles S. Whitney, *Bridges, A Study in Their Art, Science and Evolution*, New York, William Edwin Rudge, 1929. The photograph of the Canyon Diablo Bridge in Arizona, on what was then the Atlantic and Pacific Railroad, is reproduced from an original in the historical files of the Santa Fe Railway. The ironwork was fabricated by the Central Bridge Works in Buffalo, New York, and shipped to the site for assembly.

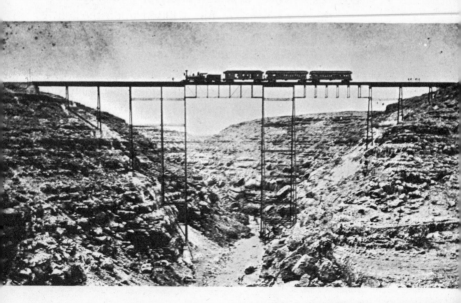

block on block, sustaining the trough through which water once flowed. But the bridge's trusses gather up and direct the forces set in motion by the trains which the structure quite literally "carries" across the canyon.

Anyone who looks at the Canyon Diablo bridge with eyes accustomed to the forms and proportions of traditional Western European construction will feel a disparity between the apparent fragility of its members and its demonstrable capacity to bear weight. An architecture based on the scheme of forms the bridge embodies would disappoint all the expectations which Western architecture has ratified for centuries. For the disposition of mass, in architecture, has traditionally conformed to what Geoffrey Scott' called our sense of "powerfully adjusted weight."* Architecture, indeed, has selected for emphasis those suggestions of pressure and resistance which, as Scott says, clearly answer to our "habitual body experience" of weight, pressure, and resistance.

Since a scheme of forms based upon the tensile strength of steel does not answer to this internal sense of physical security and strength, we cannot enjoy it, Scott insists, even if we can understand intellectually why the structure does not collapse as our eyes convince us it should. "We have no knowledge in ourselves," he says, "of any such paradoxical relations. Our aesthetic reactions are limited by our power to recreate in ourselves, imaginatively, the

* My quotations from Scott are to be found in his eloquent study of *The Architecture of Humanism.*

physical conditions suggested by the form we see."

This so-called "humanistic" conception, of architecture as an art which projects into concrete, three-dimensional form the image of our bodily sensations, movements, and moods, would necessarily exclude all structures based upon the system of tension embodied in the Canyon Diablo bridge. But many structures embodying a scheme of forms in tension do, in fact, give genuine aesthetic delight—including, most notably perhaps, the great suspension bridges of our time. One suspects that Scott's elaborate thesis is in essence only a subtly conceived justification of a long-established "custom in the eye."

The science of the modern engineer, which evolved the unprecedented structural webs of tension and compression, is like nature in that it requires from objects only such security and strength as are in fact necessary. One has only to think of the spider's web or the sunflower's stalk to realize the truth of Scott's observation that the world of nature is full of objects which are strong in ways other than those which we are habitually conscious of in our own bodies. But although there is an order in nature which the scientist can comprehend, it is not, according to Scott, an order which can be grasped by the naked eye. It is not "humanized."

There is an implication here that the eye of science—what we can "see" with the aid of photomicrographs, X rays, stroboscopic cameras, microscopes, and so on—is not "human" vision, and that human life, and the arts which express its signifi-

cance, are alike alien not only to science but to nature itself. It may be so, but there is much in the vernacular which argues the contrary, and much to suggest that the technological forms which are a part of that vernacular can beget a new "custom of the eye." We would do well, therefore, to set against this concept one which was expressed by a Tennessee architect named Harrison Gill.*

What distinguishes all truly modern architecture from all architecture of the past is, Gill argues, the very fact that it does not rely on compression alone, but employs tension as well. By its use of tension it "comes closer to the forces and mechanics of nature than ever before . . . The ability of a stalk of corn to stand erect lies in the tensile strength of its outer layers. Man and beast can move and work because of the elastic tension of tendon and sinew. All living things exist in a state of constant tension. . . . All truly modern building is alive."

Here, then, from vernacular roots a scheme of forms has evolved which is capable of expressing a humanism which takes man's mind as well as his body, his knowledge as well as his feelings, as its standard of reference, a humanism which sees man not as a stranger trying to assert his permanence in the midst of nature's inhuman and incomprehensible flux, but as a sentient part of nature's universal process.

* In his article, "What Makes Architecture Modern?", *Harper's Magazine,* July 1953.

Up Tails All*

THE THEORY
OF THE DETROIT BUSTLE

* This essay is a revision of a paper delivered as the keynote address at the International Design Conference in Aspen, Colorado, June 23, 1957, subsequently published without the author's knowledge or consent in *Arts and Architecture*, March 1958.

WORDS ARE A POOR MEDIUM in which to communicate ideas about design. Discussions of design,
by laymen or professionals, have to be carried on in
terms of verbal symbols, but verbal symbols are almost absolutely incapable of communicating any
precise or exact conception about tactile or visual
experience. If any of us tried, with words alone, to
describe precisely the difference between the 1957
and 1960 Cadillac, we would find ourselves hope-
lessly enmeshed in a clutter of words, which no one
else would have the patience to listen to and from
which no one who was not already visually acquainted with the two cars could possibly get anything but the most blurred and inaccurate sense of
what the two cars look like.

Anyone who reads what designers and critics of
design have said at various times in the past soon
becomes aware that words such as *function, structure, simplicity,* and *elegance* are so imprecise as
to be meaningless. A book published in 1877 about
the *Industrial Art* which had been exhibited at the
Centennial Exhibition in Philadelphia the year before, reads as if it might have been written by a

165

fairly advanced (if somewhat coy) twentieth-century critic, with its condemnation of showy and flashy objects, "overloaded with meaningless ornament," and its praise of "true honesty in construction, fitness of ornament to material, and decorative subordination." But when one looks at the illustrations of the objects which are praised in these terms, it is perfectly clear that the words "honesty in construction" and "fitness of ornament to material" were verbal symbols of an actuality which does not resemble what we would symbolize by those words. I think especially of a huge piece of furniture, a vast mirror frame with pedestal, carved out of wood by an Italian craftsman in imitation of ruined stonework, with broken columns, a crumbling entablature, chipped statues, and a bas-relief frieze, all overgrown with carved wooden vines in which carved birds disport themselves. The devout carver has even contrived to represent places on the massive base of his creation, where thin slabs of plaster have flaked off of what had pretended to be solid blocks of (presumably) marble, revealing the (carved) brick and mortar on which the (carved) fake masonry had really been constructed. In other words, a man who seriously admired what he verbally symbolized as "honesty in construction" and "fitness of ornament to material" could—in 1877 at least—praise an object which was a wooden imitation of a plaster and brick imitation of masonry.

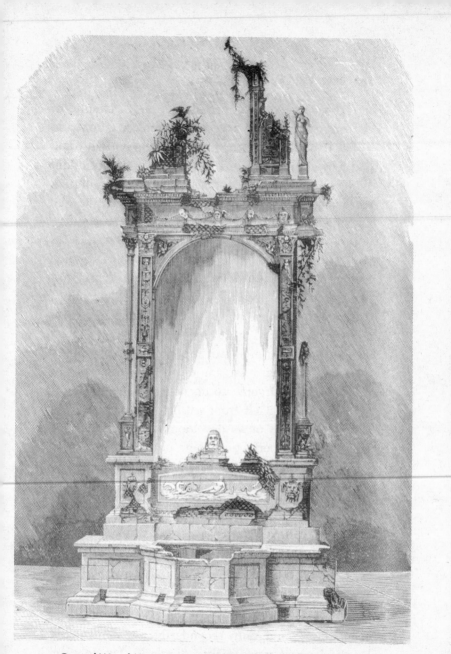

Carved Wood Mirror Frame, exhibited in the Italian Court of the Centennial International Exhibition at Philadelphia, 1876 (wood engraving reproduced from Walter Smith, *Industrial Art*—Volume II of *The Masterpieces of the Centennial International Exhibition*, Philadelphia, Gebbie & Barrie, [1877]).

It would be easy to multiply such examples of the imprecision of the verbal symbols we apply to visual experiences. But, besides being visually and tactilely imprecise, words as symbols are peculiarly subject to changing contexts. The whole group of word symbols clustering about the concept of the machine—a concept of great importance to contemporary design—provides striking evidence of this. As an illustration, take the famous passage in which Samuel Taylor Coleridge defined organic form. In a lecture on Shakespeare, given in 1818, he made a distinction between what he called mechanic form and organic form. Form is mechanic, he said, "when on any given material we impress a predetermined form, not necessarily arising out of the properties of the material." Organic form, on the other hand, is innate; shaping itself from within, as it develops, so that "the fulness of its development is one and the same with the perfection of its outward form."

We are all so used to this formulation, or to echoes of it in hundreds of later writers, that we are not likely to wonder why Coleridge used the word "mechanic" as the verbal symbol for the antithesis to "organic." Actually, the adjective "mechanic" like the noun "machine" had strongly disagreeable overtones in 1818. For one thing, it still carried its eighteenth-century meaning, defined in Dr. Johnson's great *Dictionary* as first, "mean, servile, of mean occupation," and only secondarily as "constructed by the laws of mechanicks." Similarly, Dr. Johnson

defined a mechanic (i.e., one who works according to the laws of mechanics) as "a manufacturer; a low workman." By 1818, however, the word had taken on still more disagreeable overtones, thanks to the horrors accompanying the industrial revolution. Only five years before, in 1813, the leaders of the violent Luddite anti-machine riots had stood trial in Yorkshire, and only one year earlier, in 1818, Mary Shelley had mesmerized the reading public with Frankenstein's monster—the symbol of the machine as master and destroyer of its creator. To Coleridge and his contemporaries, therefore, and to many since his time, the verbal symbol "mechanic" seemed appropriate as a contrast with "organic" because it had connotations not only of meanness and servility, but also of inhuman power, of anti-life.

The All but Celestial Mechanics

We need not trace here the subsequent ramifications of this idea. We are all aware of the prevalence of the notion that the machine is the enemy of life, and of man. All I need point out is that in the field of design, the effects of Coleridge's verbal symbol are unfortunate. There is no reason why machine-made products should be any less organic in form than those made by hand. Nothing could be more "mechanic," in Coleridge's sense, than the hand-carved Italian mirror frame I just described; both the carved frame itself and the pseudo-masonry

architecture it counterfeited are horrendous examples of predetermined form imposed upon material without regard to the material's properties. Yet there has been an anti-mechanical bias in much discussion of design ever since Coleridge's time. People of education and refinement, the vast majority of those who have run our museums and taught in our schools and colleges—the custodians, in short, of the cultivated tradition in our society—have retained the anti-machine bias inherent in the verbal symbols which Coleridge quite understandably used in 1818, but instead of which, at a different moment in history or in another social context, he might well have chosen some other word, such as "arbitrary" or "dead."

In opposition to the cultivated tradition, however, there has been, in the United States especially, for well over a century, a vernacular tradition in which the machine has been unself-consciously and enthusiastically accepted. In this tradition, the word "mechanic" has had connotations very different from those it had for Dr. Johnson and Coleridge. As early as 1843, Horatio Greenough, in one of the essays which provided the first full statement of an organic democratic aesthetic as applied to design, pointed out that it was America's mechanics, not its artists (of whom he, by the way, was one), who had discovered, in designing ships, machines, scaffolding, and bridges, the basic principle of organic design, a principle which (anticipating Louis Sullivan) he

phrased as "the unflinching adaptation of form to function." And twelve years later, in 1855, one of the most extraordinary and most neglected men in our intellectual history, Thomas Ewbank, published an astonishing volume entitled *The World a Workshop; or, the Physical Relationship of Man to Earth,* in which mechanism is envisioned as the type of God's creation—not just in the eighteenth-century sense of Celestial Mechanics, but in the sense that everything in and on the earth and in the heavens is made up of the same elements which carpenters, smiths, and other artificers work in, and that it is man's first and last duty to work with matter according to the laws of mechanics, thus imitating his Creator. Men speak of "the Architecture of the Heavens" and of God as the Great Architect, because, Ewbank says, these terms are "more in unison with current ideas of respectability" than terms like mechanics and mechanician. But they do so wrongly, because "with the works of architects we necessarily associate ideas of fixedness and immobility, while motion and change of place are essential characteristics of the universe. It is a display of forces and motions—there is nothing at rest." To control these forces, to manipulate matter, was man's reason for being, and of all men it was the mechanics, he maintained, who worked most intimately with the very stuff in which God revealed his nature and purpose.

No doubt few of those who designed or worked

with machines in nineteenth-century America, or elsewhere, consciously held such exalted notions of mechanics as did Ewbank, even though his work as U. S. Commissioner of Patents and as an active member of the Franklin Institute, together with his voluminous writings, gave him much broader influence than our historians have realized. But, whatever their notions may have been, men like Eli Whitney, Oliver Evans, Elisha King Root, George Corliss, and William Sellers evolved mechanical forms which were as "organic" in the Coleridgeian sense as any ever designed in the tradition of handcraft.

The history of design in America, as I have tried to show elsewhere,* is essentially the product of dynamic tensions between the cultivated and vernacular traditions. Ironically, the cultivated tradition, whose patrons have by and large been uninterested in, or downright contemptuous of, the machine, has been chiefly responsible for inspiring and patronizing those forms which Coleridge labeled "mechanic," while the vernacular, evolved by men who were often mechanics working with machines, has produced those contemporary forms which are most truly organic.

This is not to say that all machine-made objects are organic, or that all handmade objects are mechanic; the interaction of the cultivated and ver-

* *Made in America,* Doubleday & Co., Garden City, 1948. Re-issued in 1957 by Charles T. Branford Co., Newton Centre, Mass.

nacular traditions is more subtle and complicated than that. It is only to say that the worst machine-made objects are those whose designers have been most awed by the prestige of the cultivated tradition, just as some of the worst handmade objects have been those whose designers made foolish concessions to a hot-house-cultivated "aesthetic of the machine."

The fact that cultivated forms have influenced vernacular forms is familiar to all who have seen nineteenth-century locomotives with Gothic or Palladian windows in the cabs, and stationary steam engines whose framing is done with Doric or Corinthian columns. Less often noticed are the examples of the reverse influence of vernacular forms upon objects designed in the cultivated tradition. It is especially easy to overlook these because, in recent years, the vocabulary of designers and critics has been optimistically overeager to blur distinctions between the two traditions.

For an instructive example of the vernacular's influence on the cultivated tradition, we might look again at the spring-steel cantilever chair which Mies van der Rohe designed in 1927. The two basic elements in this design were the cantilever principle (which Mart Stam, of Holland, had used in a chair he designed the previous year) and the spring principle of bent steel. Both of these principles had been used in seats long before, but only in those vernacular areas where "artistic" effect was not consciously attended to. As Mart Stam himself said, he

found the suggestion for his original cantilever chair in the folding jump seats used in seven-passenger American automobiles. As for the spring-steel principle, it had been used for eighty years or more on the cantilevered seats of American agricultural machines (combined, incidentally, with a seat which was functionally shaped to fit the human fundament in its pear-shaped, seated position).

All this has been noted before. But what I, at least, overlooked till now is that both of the vernacular designs were functional, while the Mies van der Rohe design—so widely hailed as a masterpiece of functionalism—was not. Both the jump seat and the mower seat were functional cantilevers, because back legs on the jump seat would have interfered with the feet of the passengers sitting behind them, and there was no part of the mower to support back legs for its seat, which was cantilevered out over empty space so that the operator could sit behind the cutter bar and see what it was cutting. As for the spring effect in the mower seat, it provided a functional shock absorber on a rough-riding machine. For household chairs, however, which are used on relatively flat surfaces which don't jounce, neither the cantilever nor the spring was quite relevant. The Mies van der Rohe design was, fundamentally, pure playfulness—the product of cultivated aesthetic playing solemnly with forms developed in the vernacular.

Off Again, on Again, Fins Again

In recent years, since about 1930, the prestige of genuine vernacular forms has enormously increased, partly as a result of social and economic forces which, during the depression, made economy and simplicity attractive, and partly because in those years certain vernacular forms (especially those of the airplane) reached a degree of refinement which gave them an unimpeachable appropriateness and made them a source of liberated delight. Aerodynamic forms have, in fact, acquired an authority as classically absolute as the sculptural forms of Periclean Athens, the blank verse dramatic forms of Elizabethan England, or the choral forms of eighteenth-century Germany. And, as Dr. Jacob Bronowski said, in a speech published in *Industrial Design,* because these vernacular designs (he calls them pioneer designs) interest and satisfy us, "there grows from them a custom in the eye" which forms our taste in other fields as well. We like to design and to buy streamlined toasters and irons not (as Dr. Bronowski sensibly points out) because we have any expectation of their flying, but because machines that fly have taught us to question protuberant decoration and to admire streamlined forms. To me it seems likely that it is to this magnetic appeal, rather than to the Freudian symbolism in which some critics are so artlessly absorbed, that we owe

the rocket-shaped ornaments and tail fins of contemporary Detroit.

I am convinced that if we could really determine why the designers designed those tail fins, and
why the car-buying public liked them, we could
clear up some of the confusions which befuddle
many of our opinions and judgments about contemporary design. In this connection, I am reminded of
an idea I encountered in Don Wallance's book,
Shaping America's Products, which may serve as a
useful text for further discussion. Mr. Wallance
distinguishes at one point between objects whose
inner structure and outer form are integral—such as
a pottery bowl or a plywood chair—and, on the
other hand, objects whose outer forms merely
sheath an inner structure or mechanism—objects
such as refrigerators or radios, whose essential nature
separates the process of making from the process of
designing. Like all verbal classifications, these are
useful only so long as we stay in the middle of
them, keeping clear of the peripheries where the
distinctions become blurred. But, if we do stay in
the middle, we can, I think, get a helpful perspective
on those much-maligned fins and on other controversial aspects of design.

When we consider objects whose inner structure and outer form are integral—such as a tea cup
or a glass tumbler—it seems to me that we can all,
designers and consumers alike, agree upon what
constitutes good design. We can without too much

176

difficulty determine whether the design is appropriate to the tools with which it is made, to the materials of which it is made, and to the uses for which it is made; whether it has evolved from the inner structure; in short, whether it is organic and functional.

In considering objects of the other class, whose outer forms merely sheath an inner structure which designer and public agree should be covered up—such as an eighteenth-century grandfather clock, or a twentieth-century toaster—we are, however, in an area where the question of the appropriateness of the design becomes much more complicated, becomes, in fact, not a matter of logic, but of taste. And we may as well define taste, right now, as that sort of preference for one or another form which is relevant only when form is independent of function. Or, to put it differently, taste is that sort of form-preference which can logically be illogical, and usually is. Taste can have little to do with the design of an airplane wing or a propeller blade, but almost everything to do with the design of a refrigerator cabinet or a woman's dress.

It was, I think, to the failure to distinguish between these two classes of objects that Raymond Loewy was objecting when he said some years ago that he couldn't go along with those critics who brand the shell or wrapper treatment as a breach of design integrity. If so, I heartily agree with him. But, in making his counter-argument, Mr. Loewy seems to me to have reinforced the confusion instead

of clearing it up. An airplane, he pointed out, is ~~internally a complex arrangement (I think he said~~ messy) of gadgets, wiring, tubes, dials, ducts, spars, levers, rivets, and controls. Everything is functionally correct, but it would look extremely confusing if it showed. It is only the airplane's skin, or shell, Mr. Loewy maintains, which by covering this internal confusion makes the airplane a form of such elegance. And from this he concludes that "when a given product has been reduced to its functional best and still looks disorganized and ugly, a plain, simple shield . . . is aesthetically justified." This shield, he argues, becomes functional, "the specific function being to eliminate confusion."*

Now, much as I admire Mr. Loewy's plain and simply shielded locomotives and several other designs of his, I think it is worth pointing out that he is cheating in this passage; because the skin of an airplane is not a simple shield at all; it *is* the airplane; it *is* the organic structural form of the object, into which all those gadgets, tubes, dials, and ducts must be stuffed as neatly as may be. It is not, like a refrigerator shell or a clock case, something which can be one shape or another, fussy or plain, angular or rounded, according to the designer's or the consumer's whim. Mr. Loewy happens to have (or at least had when he wrote his book) a taste for non-angular simplicity. Elsewhere in the book he lays

* *Never Leave Well Enough Alone,* Simon & Schuster, New York, 1951.

it down as a law of design that "the general mass [of an object] should be flowing, graceful, free of sharp corners and brutal radii"—which, of course, is not a law of design at all, but merely a manifesto of taste, and one to which some very eminent designers, including the designer of the Pyramids, and Sir Charles Eastlake, and Mies van der Rohe, to name some diverse examples, would not have subscribed.

I happen to prefer Mr. Loewy's designs to those of Sir Charles Eastlake. All I am trying to point out is that there is a difference between the skin of an airplane and the shield or sheath which covers an automobile engine or a toaster mechanism, and that it is useful to avoid confusing the two. To justify the hood of an auto engine by analogy with the nacelle of a plane tells us something about the contemporary prestige of aerodynamic form, but nothing at all about what good design of an automobile is.

Think again of the Cadillac's famous (or infamous) fins, or of their exuberant progeny on other cars. In Don Wallance's terms, these forms are sheaths, in no sense integral with the inner structure or mechanism of the car; and as I have suggested, there is no reason why they shouldn't be sheaths, or why we should try to apply to them, or to any other sheath design, the criteria we apply to integral designs. They are not functional, in Greenough's sense, nor organic in Coleridge's, and it strikes me

as silly for the advertisements to try to pretend they are. I am convinced those fins are the shape they are primarily because some designer liked their looks, and because a good many car buyers (*not* including me) agree with him. I am also convinced that both the designer and the buyer like the look because the fins echo forms which were functionally evolved in aerodynamics and are therefore pleasing.

If we are going to use the term functional in our discussion of design, let us agree that it has two quite different meanings, one of which applies to integral design, and one of which applies to sheath design. One kind of functionalism has to do with the appropriateness of design to tools, material, and use, and tends toward simplification and what Greenough calls "the majesty of the essential." The other

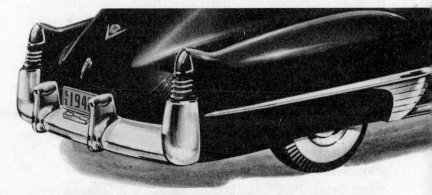

The prototypical "tail fins." Detail of the 1948 Cadillac (photograph courtesy of General Motors Photographic Section).

180

kind of functionalism has to do less with the structure of the object than with the structure of the designer's and the consumers' psyches, and tends whimsically toward the simple or the baroque, depending on lots of things which we needn't here be concerned about. To keep it separate from the other sort of functionalism, why don't we simply and honestly label it effective packaging?

Most features of automobile design, or "styling," as it is more significantly called, like most features of toaster design and dress design, are packaging in precisely the sense that the wrapper for a bar of candy and the box for cereal are packaging. The couturier's bustle and the Detroit car stylist's bustle are to be judged by the same standards, and effective packaging does have its own standards (some of which, of course, are utilitarian) which merit serious and respectful attention in their own right, undiluted by carry-overs from integral design. It seems to me that the sooner we all—designers and public alike—stop confusing the two, the sooner we will be able to agree upon what we are talking about in our discussions of design.

Those tail fins are as "functional" as the shape of a bomber's wing, though their function is less utilitarian. They have, of course, some utilitarian functions. They do hold the taillights up high, where they are more visible than taillights used to be in traffic, and they are said to serve some aerodynamic function at high speeds. But their chief function

was to delight the eye and attract buyers, which is the principal function of all packaging in our economy. This they did, superlatively well. The fact that some of us had other ideas about what a suitable package for the rear end of a car should be proved only how wrong we were.

We were wrong, I think, because we persisted in thinking of automobiles as pure vernacular designs. Most of us who disparaged the tail fins were admirers of the army jeep and its early civilian counterpart, whose design frankly acknowledged that it was a four-wheeled vehicle with a motor up front. In this respect the jeep was a direct descendant of the Model-T Ford, solidly based in the vernacular: a mechanical form which was almost wholly "organic" in Coleridge's sense.

The finned Cadillac, on the other hand, was a sheath design. Coleridge would have called it "mechanic," in the sense that the fins and other elements of the design were "predetermined" forms imposed upon the material. But as I have tried to show, this does not mean that the Cadillac sheath was non-functional. It means only that the function it served was non-utilitarian, having more to do with the psychological uses of an automobile than with mechanical transportation.

What we must not overlook, if we are interested in American developments in design, is that the predetermined "mechanic" forms employed in this tremendously successful and influential sheath de-

sign were not borrowed from the pre-industrial handcraft tradition. They were borrowed from another area of design rooted in the vernacular: from the airplane, which even more than the automobile, epitomizes the concern with motion and mobility in our technological civilization. Like almost everything designed in our culture, those finned Cadillacs are a product of the dynamic tensions between vernacular and cultivated influences. But it is a mark of how far we have come since the Centennial's ornate pedestaled mirror frame that the "cultivated" forms here applied to an object which emerged from the vernacular are forms which had themselves been developed and refined from other vernacular sources. Our vernacular, in some areas at least, has become a cultivated tradition of our own.

Soft Sell, Hard Sell,
Padded Sell*

* This essay, in slightly different form, was written to be read at the University of Michigan, May 13, 1960, as one of a series of University Lectures, by various speakers, on Advertising in American Society.

A FEW WEEKS AGO I saw a television commercial which showed a man—an "ordinary Joe," a you-and-me sort of fellow, with loosened tie and unbuttoned collar—looking at television commercials. A voice in the background, accounting for the man's changing expressions of dismay, explained that the man was watching a series of commercials for various brands of cigarettes, each of which promised him some special delight. We were not shown the various commercials he was watching; we saw only his face and body as he reacted to them. Finally he saw a new commercial, advertising a new brand of cigarette which combined all the virtues of the other brands. His face relaxed; he smiled contentedly and sank back in his overstuffed chair; and the announcer's voice said, "Lucky Joe! He doesn't have to watch the commercials any more."

The implications of this filmed advertisement seemed to me to be interesting. What is going on in the advertising business when an advertisement implies that one merit of the product is that, having discovered it, you don't have to look at advertise-

ments any more? My interest was further aroused when I discovered, some days later, that this particular commercial had won a top award in the industry's own annual competition sponsored by the Art Directors' Club. Are we faced with the possibility that the advertising men are getting self-conscious about how boring some of their advertisements are? Is it possible that the trade is even more bored by a good deal of what it is doing than the audience is?

If this particular TV commercial were an isolated phenomenon, it might not be important. But it strikes me that there are a number of recent ads which reflect an amused disenchantment with the tenor of advertising in general. I think, for instance, of Bert and Harry Piel and their irreverent mockery of stale advertising techniques; of a Kaiser Foil ad, cast in the form of a burlesque soap opera; and of a job-wanted ad which ran in the New York *Times* recently, in which a young woman, looking for a job as a copy writer in an advertising agency, began her appeal with: "Soft sell, hard sell, padded sell. From Paris frocks to cuckoo clocks . . . you name it. I've done it, proud!" And one has only to read the editorials, and the letters from readers, in such a trade publication as *Advertising Age* to be aware of how much earnest and responsible self-criticism the advertising men engage in.

In looking at advertising as an aspect of American culture, I am functioning as a non-expert. My

knowledge of the business is limited to the impact its products have upon me and my friends and acquaintances, and to what I have picked up unsystematically from a few friends who are in various branches of the business and from desultory reading about it. I have not read any of the best-selling books which, I gather, have exposed the inner workings of Madison Avenue, and I have only glanced at such scholarly studies as Neil Borden's *Advertising in Our Economy*. My approach, then, is that of an interested observer of the American scene, without special inside knowledge of the advertising business.

Like most people I know, I have a nostalgic fondness for the ads I grew up on and the sediment of phrases and pictures which remains from them in my memory: the elegant lines of the 1917 Locomobile touring car on the back cover of *Harper's Magazine;* the Coles Philips "Holeproof Hosiery" girls; W. L. Douglas "pegging shoes at the age of seven"; and such phrases as "not even her best friends would tell her . . ." and "too late for Herpicide." Like most people I know, I am likely to find the advertisements in some contemporary magazines more interesting, visually and verbally, than the editorial matter surrounding them. Like most people I know, I feel insulted by the absurd TV posturing of widemouthed men who hold up cigarette packs or cake mixes and point to the letters on the box as they read them to me, and by the

inane posturing of waxen girls with slick smiles caressing refrigerators and washing machines. Like most people I know, I think it is dismaying if people can in effect be forced, by the irrational emotional appeal of advertising, to buy what they do not really want or need; and also, like most people I know, I am sure that neither I nor anyone I know is so naïve as to be unduly affected by such irrational factors. It is just everybody else who falls for the stuff.

It was David Riesman and his collaborators in *The Lonely Crowd* who first suggested, I think, that advertising may be essentially "a fantastic fraud, presenting an image of America taken seriously by no one, least of all by the advertising men who create it." By ripping the suggestion out of the context of Riesman's argument as a whole, I deprive it of its subtlety; but the skeptical attitude it suggests is perhaps a healthy one in which to begin our consideration of a subject about which many of us have firm but conflicting opinions. There are, at any rate, some startling data which suggest that advertising is not quite doing the job it pretends to be doing (and which its impassioned critics too readily give it credit for). A recent survey by Trendex, the TV rating service, indicated that less than twenty per cent of those who watch the popular "Peter Gunn" show know what products the show is sponsored by and that a quarter of those who watch "Alcoa Presents" don't know who sponsors it.

Soft Sell, Hard Sell, Padded Sell

The field of advertising is so broad, there are so many kinds of advertisements, with so little in common, that we should limit our discussion in some way. When I think about advertising, I think chiefly in terms of those ads in which picture and text are combined in a layout whose effectiveness depends upon its qualities as a design. But what of the television commercial? What of billboards, and the neon signs which lure us into bars and grills? What of radio commercials, and of the classified ads which constitute such a large proportion of the total advertising in our newspapers? Are the things that may be said of the ads on television equally true of the Classified ads in Sunday's New York *Times?* Which is more significant of our culture: the ads in the current issue of *McCall's,* or the strange mélange in *The Old Farmer's Almanac,* with its glossy insert of double-page color spreads offering *Chiquita Banana's Cookbook,* side by side with crudely illustrated ads with chatty text offering rupture-easers, gladiolus bulbs, and aromatic fish bait, plus a number of ads, mostly in very small type, beginning, "Are you growing too old too fast?" or, "I nearly itched to death for 7½ years," and so on?

Do we lump all these together when we think about advertising as an institution in our society? Or do we merely select, out of the confused welter of different types of advertising, those which our prejudices happen to be excited by? I raise these

questions not because I intend to be systematic, but merely as a warning that my generalizations should be tested against a variety of types of advertising, some of which have little in common with the others.

The Ads as Potter's Field

My concern about advertising is a double one. I am concerned about the role the institution plays in our society, and I am concerned about the quality of the advertisements it produces. And since the quality of advertisements must be judged in terms of the function which they serve, let us begin by trying to clarify our notions about what the role of advertising is.

No one who speculates about advertising as an institution can overlook the chapter on advertising in Professor David Potter's book, *People of Plenty*, which grew out of his Walgreen Foundation lectures in 1954. And since one encounters frequent references to this chapter in the comments of professional advertising men as well as elsewhere, references which suggest a widespread acceptance of the analysis it presents, we should consider Professor Potter's argument.

Professor Potter discusses advertising as the characteristic institution of a society based upon an economy of abundance. Advertising, he argues, would never have been a very significant force in an economy of scarcity, because if there is less than

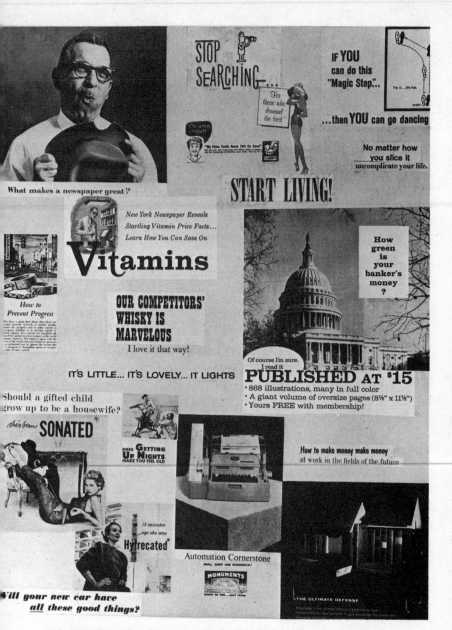

A Confusion of Different Types of Ads (confused by the author).

enough food, clothing, or transportation to satisfy the demand, all that is needed is the mere announcement of what products are available, and where. But when supply outstrips demand, when there is abundance, the role of advertising changes to one of influencing consumer tastes and creating consumer demand. In a consumer-oriented society, such as ours, he says, the only institution capable of educating people to *be* consumers is advertising.

Professor Potter therefore ranks advertising as one of the basic institutions of social control—and the only one which has come into existence directly and wholly in response to the needs of a consumer society. What distinguishes advertising from such traditional institutions of social control as the church and education, in Professor Potter's view, is that there is in its dynamics

> . . . no motivation to seek the improvement of the individual or to impart qualities of social usefulness, unless conformity to material values may be so characterized. And though it wields an immense social influence, comparable to the influence of religion and learning, it has no social goals and no social responsibility for what it does with its influence, so long as it refrains from palpable violations of truth and decency.

It is this social irresponsibility, this lack of any social purpose to balance its social power, which Professor Potter sees as the basic cause for concern

about the role of advertising as an institution. He is not unduly troubled by the occasional breaches of taste or deviations from sound ethical conduct which stain the record; one gathers that he would not join those who converted the recent quiz-show and payola scandals into justifications for blanket condemnation of advertising. But neither is he overly impressed by the fairly frequent examples of what he calls "high-minded types of advertising"—the types, one supposes, which are annually applauded by the *Saturday Review*'s awards "for distinguished advertising in the public interest." Neither sort is intrinsic to the institution of advertising as such, he says. What *is* intrinsic, as Potter sees it, is the fact that advertising "regards man as a consumer and defines its own mission as one of stimulating him to consume or to desire to consume."

This might not be bad, one gathers, were it not for the fact that the institution of advertising has a controlling influence in the mass-media: magazines, newspapers, radio, television, and so on. Because of advertising's influence, Professor Potter argues, the mass-media are permeated with efforts to stimulate and exploit "materialistic drives and emulative anxieties" and to validate, sanction, and standardize these drives and anxieties "as accepted criteria of social value."

You may have noticed that Professor Potter is alarmed at the existence of a powerful institution which is not self-conscious about its role as a

guardian of social values, which does not seek to "improve" the individual or to "impart qualities of social usefulness." The implication of this alarm, it seems to me, is that the drives and anxieties of the consumer (those drives and anxieties which advertising allegedly stimulates and exploits) are "bad" things and are the result of "wrong" values. Advertising, one gathers, should use its power to change these values and to induce other drives (and, presumably, other anxieties).

For myself, I rather like the idea that modern industrial civilization—this society of abundance in which we live—has produced one institution which, unlike those which survive from earlier and different eras, makes no assumpton that those who control its powerful resources have the duty or the right to impose their values upon the rest of us. Of course I know that individual advertisers do try to use the institution for their own ends, and in support of their particular values. Labor unions sponsor news commentators who are favorable to the union cause and who select and slant the news in their interest, just as a famous machine-tool company runs a full-page ad in national magazines headed "Shouldn't a worker's son have a strike vote, too?" in which it is argued that however a strike comes out, the worker's children will suffer. But the institution of advertising is not committed to imposing a certain set of values and standards upon society; its job is to discover, and appeal to, the changing values and standards

which those who live in our society are constantly evolving for themselves. If an advertiser summons up courage enough to assert his own values, he asserts them at his own risk; because, if a considerable number of his prospective customers are offended by his views, they will not respond to his appeal. There are emotional boycotts as well as economic ones.

I do not want to oversimplify here. I am aware that there are techniques, both pictorial and verbal, for creating an irrelevantly favorable aura around ideas as well as products. I know that, from the point of view of sheer logic, there is no reason to travel by jet because an advertisement associates jets with our hopes for the future by showing the disarming rear view of a little boy looking out of what the small type tells you is one of "the DC-8's big picture windows—twice the size of those in other jets." I know that there is no reason to buy a certain brand of sheets because an ad shows them flapping on a clothesline behind a bosomy girl, hanging her largely uncovered attractions over a fence as she tells a male neighbor, "There's not a wrinkle in them, so I think I'll let them wave in the breeze all afternoon." But I also know that there is no reason to buy a particular container because the advertisement associates it with modern art and the great ideas of Western man. Furthermore, I do not imagine that either little boys, or the female breast, or the

great ideas of Western man are valued either more or less because of the ads.

There is obviously room for all sorts of conflicting opinions about specific advertisements, specific advertising campaigns, and specific policies in the advertising business. But many of the charges brought against advertising are, it seems to me, charges which should properly be brought against society as a whole. We cannot examine contemporary advertisements as clues to the secret dreams of mass-man, as Herbert Marshall McLuhan has done in his book *The Mechanical Bride,* on the assumption that they are successful because they appeal to certain emotional values which mass-man holds dear, and then turn things about and argue that mass-man holds these values dear because the ads have taught him to do so. The advertising agencies, Mr. McLuhan says, "express for the collective society that which dreams and uncensored behavior do in individuals," but in the next breath he tells us that the agencies, like Hollywood, "are always trying to get inside the public mind in order to impose their collective dreams on that inner stage."

The confusion which underlies McLuhan's analysis—and a good deal of similar criticism of advertising—is related, I think, to a confusion which is evident in Professor Potter's analysis. He classifies advertising as "an institution of social control" comparable to education and the church, and at the same time defines it as an institution which has

"no social goals." We can all agree, to be sure, that advertising has considerable influence in our society, but if it has "no social goals" it is hard to see how it can be classed as an institution of social control.

If advertising is, by definition, an institution which came into existence and developed its techniques solely to stimulate people "to consume or to desire to consume," how can we rationally judge its performance by standards which apply only to the work of institutions seeking to improve the individual or "to impart qualities of social usefulness"? We can, of course, lament the fact that an institution of the sort ever came into existence, but this amounts to little more than a wish that the world were not as it is. If we do not like the world which advertising reflects, let us by all means do what we can to change it, but let us not suppose that we can change it by smashing the mirror.

If advertising is the characteristic institution of an economy of abundance, our wish that it more nearly resembled institutions inherited from an economy of scarcity may be wistfully understandable. The wish is unlikely, however, to suggest appropriate standards by which to judge the institution's performance. The products of an institution whose function it is to stimulate consumption should be judged by their success in achieving that end, not by their failure to do other things, however worthy those other things may be in themselves.

The Goods or the Good?

Conflicting views on this subject probably account for much of the contemporary disagreement about what a good advertisement is. For example, none of the medals or certificates of merit awarded in the Art Directors' Club's 1960 competition went to advertisements which received that year's *Saturday Review* awards for distinguished advertising. In the Art Directors' Club's competition advertisements are judged by standards of creative excellence in design. The *Saturday Review* awards committee selects advertisements according to standards of "the public interest"—as that interest is conceived by a board of distinguished educators, editors, publishers, and business executives. The ads which seem best to one group do not seem best to the other, because one group is judging primarily in terms of the message the ads convey and the other is judging primarily in terms of the techniques by which the messages are conveyed.

There is, of course, no necessary incompatibility between creative design and the public interest, though those in charge of the traditional institutions of social control sometimes act as though they thought there were. In architectural design, for instance, the creative developments of the late nineteenth and early twentieth century, which underlie the best work of our own period, emerged in such

vernacular areas as amusement parks and industrial plants and were shunned by the churches and universities until, in the normal course of things, they had become themselves traditional and the genuine creators had gone on to other things.

The values of good design, it seems to me, are more appropriate to our judgment of advertisements than those of "the public interest" as defined by educators, business leaders, or public servants. If advertising, as an institution, is by its very nature committed to the view of man as a consumer who is to be encouraged to consume, advertisements surely should be judged on their effectiveness in promoting consumption. If we object, as all of us certainly do, to some of the things the ads try to persuade us to consume (whether those things be stupidly designed cars or attitudes toward labor), we should direct our disapproval toward the sponsor of the advertisement, not toward the copy writers, artists, photographers, and layout men who create the advertisements. To condemn an ad because it skillfully employs verbal and visual techniques to make cigarette smoking seem desirable, when we happen to think cigarette smoking is undesirable, is rather like condemning *Paradise Lost* because we disapprove of its theology and think we know that its cosmology is wrong.

It is interesting, nevertheless, to see how often nowadays irrelevant considerations enter into our judgment of ads, even in advertising circles. The pages of trade magazines in the field are full of

evidence that men and women in the business are convinced of the vast power of their techniques for "informing, persuading, and inspiring" and that they want to have clear consciences about their use of that power. A number of advertising executives serve on the *Saturday Review*'s committee of awards. And the Advertising Council, supported by the various advertising agencies, has endorsed and sponsored advertising campaigns in favor of better schools, cancer prevention, support of the United Nations, and other things which its members agree are socially desirable.

All this is no doubt admirable, from the point of view of those who favor better schools, cancer prevention, and the United Nations—as I, for one, do. We may, to be sure, have certain qualms if we remember that a number of thoughtful Americans have reservations about the United Nations; we may wonder whether coming out in favor of better schools serves any very useful purpose unless the emotion is attached to some specific conception of what would make the schools better; and we may wonder whether cancer prevention is better served by pleas to discover it early than by the cigarette filters which advertisements so fervently recommend to us. But in general there is something pleasant enough about having the representatives of such a prosperous institution as advertising devote some of their profits from it to the support of a collateral institution, such

as the Advertising Council, whose public gestures are obviously well intentioned.

Furthermore, one can well understand the impulse behind such gestures if one recognizes that the analogy I suggested a moment ago, between an advertisement and Milton's epic poem, is in one important respect inaccurate. The techniques of advertising, unlike the techniques of the poet, are employed to communicate someone else's message, not that of the writers, artists, and designers who create the advertisements. Men and women in advertising are the skilled masters of techniques which are—and must be, in a free society—available to all who want them and can pay for them. In this sense, their business is not unlike that of the telephone company, or of such public carriers as the railroads and airlines. An airline has no more right or obligation to determine whether it is socially desirable to transport me from New York to Michigan or Colorado than an advertising agency has to determine whether it is socially desirable to permit a manufacturer of toilet water to imply that my wife should use his product if she wants to be physically desirable to men who drive Jaguar sports cars.

Advertising, then, is rather like an art in which the techniques have, to a great extent, been divorced from subject matter. The subject matter is provided by the patron, as it were, and the execution alone is the responsibility of the artist. An advertising agency is, to some extent, like a team of poets

203

laureate with not one institutional patron but dozens, each with its own diverse interests to be served, much as if England had a team of poets laureate who had to collaborate on an ode on the merits of nationalized railways, and one on the attractions of British woolens, at the same time that they celebrated the marriage of Princess Margaret. It is a difficult position to be in—especially for people who, like the writers, artists, and designers who produce the advertisements, are by nature and temperament disposed to the lonely responsibility of creativeness. Not that the position of the creative people in advertising is unique; it is not. In the movie studios, and in the corporate journalism of *Time* and *Newsweek*, and in many other areas of contemporary life, similar problems exist. But this team creativeness which the arts grounded in modern technology seem to require presents perplexing problems, not the least of which is the divorcing of techniques from subject matter; and it is no wonder that the people involved have qualms about some of the subject matter to which they have to apply their techniques. Creative people in the visual and verbal arts often have values which are antithetical to those of people who are likely to be successful managers and entrepreneurs in industry—yet it is the leaders of industry who prescribe much of the subject matter on which advertising must employ its techniques. It is no wonder that some of those engaged in advertising, acting in response to the promptings of their individual con-

sciences, either leave the business and write savage novels about it, or work from within, as it were, to make advertising serve some values which seem to them to be "in the public interest."

But I cannot help wondering if such activities are not partly responsible for the aura of pretentiousness which has fallen like a blight on so much contemporary advertising. I may exaggerate, but it seems to me that there is a depressing amount of evidence that advertising is suffering from a sort of stuffy do-goodism, brought on by those who seek to impose upon it values which bear no relation to the dynamics of the institution itself. An institution which arose in response to the needs of a consumer-oriented economy of abundance, based upon modern technology, may have all sorts of faults; but they are not likely to be eliminated or alleviated by attempts to warp the institution into the service of values relevant to other institutions.

Do Public Interest Ads Serve the Public Interest?

Let me illustrate my point concretely. Those who object to the social irresponsibility of advertising, seem to approve heartily the series of advertisements, sponsored by the Container Corporation, which present reproductions of modern paintings in conjunction with quotations from the Bible, or *The Education of Henry Adams,* or some other repository

of what the ads call "Great Ideas of Western Man." One of the ads in this series won the top award in the 1960 *Saturday Review* competition.

This series may or may not be effective in increasing the consumption of containers. The late Walter Paepcke, who initiated the series, said it was not designed to sell boxes but to establish for his company a reputation which would in the long run bring more sales. Admen who approve of the series point to the fact that company sales have greatly increased in recent years. Others may wonder whether increased sales of boxes and containers, which are sold to other manufacturers as packages for their products, do not probably owe more to aggressive salesmen and to the proved quality of the containers than to the company's "corporate image" of itself as a patron of the arts and of man's cultural heritage. But whether or not the ads are good, by fiscal standards, they seem to be universally approved in terms of their service to "the public interest."

If we look at the ads in this series from a different point of view, however, and judge them by standards appropriate to designed layouts of picture and text, we may discover that the public interest is less well served by them than we are supposed to believe. Let us grant that the ads are designed to induce us to consume the notion that the Container Corporation of America is a good company because it believes in the Great Ideas of Western Man (a

later series, by the way, pays homage to the Great Ideas of Eastern Man as well) and also sponsors modern art. And for the sake of the argument let us grant the dubious point that it is because they have effectively induced the consumption of this notion that sales of boxes have increased. And, having made these concessions, let us examine 1960's prize-winning ad.

The "great idea" which the ad celebrates is contained in a sentence quoted in large type from Henry Adams, namely: "A teacher affects eternity; he can never tell where his influence stops." Inserted between the two lines of type which this quotation requires is a color reproduction of a painting entitled "Primeval Wall" which some very small type, running vertically along the right-hand edge of the picture, tells us "represents the ancient cave paintings where the drama of teaching began a hundred million years ago." Except for modest identifications of the source of the quote, and the artist who made the painting, and the sponsoring corporation, neatly placed at the bottom of the page, that is all there is to it.

The ad is obviously intended to appeal to the public's respect for education and for the arts, though it is difficult to see what relevance the representation of the cave painting has to the idea expressed in the quotation. Iconographically, the abstract forms in the picture make no visual communication that in any way suggests teaching, handsome

207

as they are in themselves and in their formal and tonal relationship to one another and to the space defined by the mottled, rectangular background. Nor does the explanatory vertical strip of small type explain very much, with its ambiguous reference to "cave paintings where the drama of teaching began." (Did teaching begin in the paintings or in the caves? Is there any evidence that it began in either place?) There seems to be something pretentious about the juxtaposition of the picture with the Adams text.

And what of the text? Is it in fact a great idea of Western man? Is it not true that a bartender and an operator of a turret lathe also affect eternity and can never tell where their influence stops? Granted that in the context of Adams's book the idea was significant, the isolated sentence can scarcely be called a "great idea." In fact, is there not something pretentious about the whole conception of presenting great ideas in one-sentence capsule form? Is not a great idea one which is, like Willard Gibbs's theories of thermodynamics, or Aristotle's idea about the relations of form and matter, by definition so complex that it cannot be conveyed in a single motto-like sentence?

Even so, it may be argued, the ad implies nice things about teachers, and since teachers are a Good Thing, the ad is surely in the public interest. But of course teachers aren't necessarily a good thing at all; a bad teacher is a very bad thing indeed, especially considering the fact that, like the bartender, he af-

fects eternity. So, much as I selfishly hope, being a teacher, that the prize-winning ad leads to public willingness to provide higher salaries for teachers, I am not really convinced that such a result would be in the public interest unless there were some way to insure that the higher salaries would attract good teachers, not bad ones, to the profession.

What can be said, however, about the prize-winning advertisement's contribution to the worthy cause of modern art? In considering this question we shall encounter, even more directly perhaps than in our discussion of other aspects of the ad, the criteria which seem to me to be relevant to our judgment of advertising.

On the face of it, this ad, like the others in the series, makes part of its appeal by association with contemporary painting. It uses the reproduction of a painting for "eyeappeal," for the attention-getting qualities of design which the reproduction has, and it seeks to identify the sponsoring manufacturer with certain values which the sponsor associates with modern art. As Mr. Paepcke told an interviewer from *Advertising Age* in 1955, modern art was used in the ads because "a packaging firm has to be modern." Packagers, he said, "want sleek, up-to-date material; for that reason we don't think Giotto or Gainsborough would do for us."

One may wonder what service is done to modern painting by exploiting its "sleek, up-to-date" qualities, even though one may acknowledge that

209

the fees paid to the artists whose paintings are reproduced must be as welcome to them as a raise
in salary is to a teacher. Doing good to modern
artists is not, however, the same as doing good to
modern art, any more than raising my salary is the
same as making me a better teacher.

It is sometimes argued that the cause of modern
painting is well served by making reproductions of
it so widely available, but here we come up against
the technical conditions which are involved in advertising. Magazine advertisements such as those in
the "great ideas" series are reproduced by photo-
mechanical processes. They are printed from plates
made by photoengravers, and the photoengraving
process is such that the colors in a painting are inevitably distorted unless the reproduction is precisely
the same size as the original, and unless its surface has
exactly the same texture. More than thirty years ago,
Gordon Aymar, then art director of the J. Walter
Thompson agency, protested against the use of over-
size oil paintings as the basis for advertisements in
which they have to be reduced to a sixth or an eighth
of their original size. He was, of course, thinking primarily in terms of the added difficulty which the
agency and the photoengravers had in trying to ap-
proximate the color values of the original art work.
To the agency, and the craftsmen in photoengraving,
it made more sense to employ artists to paint pictures
of appropriate size and to work in colors easily
matched by the process-inks which are used in print-

ing plants. But from the artist's point of view, also, the reproduction of a painting in reduced size is undesirable—unless one can conceive of a painting in which color values are inconsequential. In representational painting, perhaps, the iconographic elements of the design may outweigh the color relationships in interest, so that a reduced reproduction, with its inevitable color distortion, may retain the painting's principal values. But in reproductions of modern paintings the changed color values surely distort the essential qualities of the work of art.

Looked at from this point of view, the prize-winning public-interest ad appears to be less favorable to the public interest than it pretends to be. If, as there is some reason to suspect, the ad has also had little effect in stimulating the consumption of containers, either directly or indirectly through creating a favorable image of the sponsoring corporation in the minds of packagers, it is inefficient as well as pretentious.

One turns with relief to the ads which are frankly out to sell a product or a service, by associating it in picture and text with values which potential consumers are likely to admire, and which employ techniques of writing and of picture making which are appropriate to the advertising medium involved —a good photograph of the bottle or the bra. One wonders if, in the end, the public interest will not best be served, in this opulent economy of ours, by freeing the institution of advertising from pressures

to adopt values which are alien to it, and by allowing the creative, talented writers, artists, and designers in the agencies to create ads which do the job advertising can effectively do.

It would surely be in the public interest to remember that many, if not most, of our objections to advertising are really objections to some of the businesses and other institutions of social control which employ advertising as a means of competing for our attention. In a free society a wide variety of institutions will forever be engaged in such competition, and in a free society those of us who have one set of values will always be tempted to wish that those with opposing values could be silenced. The constant challenge to our cause, when those with other values have equal access to the skilled techniques of persuading and inspiring, is likely to teach us respect for what Edward Filene called "the intolerable fatigue of persuasion." The danger is that it may even persuade us that, in the interest of our particular "truth," the advertising agency's skilled techniques should be denied to those whose values we disapprove. Freedom is a fatiguing state of affairs. But I like to think, as I leaf through our contemporary magazines, with their wealth of good and not-so-good ads, that freedom is worth the fatigue.

Certainly freedom for the creative people in the advertising agencies is worth it. Most of the advertisements which have won medals in the past few years in the Art Directors' Club's competition were

produced by men and women working in small agencies, where individual creative talents are not subordinated—as they tend to be in the large agencies —to market research and the electronic computation of taste. It was one of the small, relatively new agencies which produced that television commercial I began by describing—the one which showed us the lucky Joe who wouldn't have to watch commercials any more. And the delightful thing about that ad for Alpine cigarettes is, of course, that far from making us want to stop looking at commercials, it has just the opposite effect. I will watch any Alpine commercials that come along, if they maintain such standards. I might even switch to Alpine cigarettes.

The Beer Can by the Highway;*

OR, WHATEVER BECAME OF EMERSON?

* The earliest version of this essay was written as an address to be delivered at Mills College, Oakland, California, April 4, 1957, and was published in the *Mills Quarterly*. A subsequent version was published in *Harper's Magazine*, March 1959, under the title "Waste Not, Have Not."

Two aspects of American civilization strike almost everyone: the abundance it enjoys, and the waste it permits (if it does not enjoy that too). As a London *Times* reviewer observed, in a discussion of three important books on American history, the occupation and development of this country has been "a wasteful process," and the American god "was not, is not thrifty. Nor is he, or was he, tidy."

Toward this untidy abundance the Europeans' attitude has generally been what George Nelson, the architect-designer, describes as "a blend of appalled curiosity, downright disbelief, righteous indignation, and envy." On what comprehensible basis, they want to know, can a nation "throw away its cars when the ash trays are full" and yet prosper? How, in short, can a nation get richer and richer—achieve more and more abundance—as it grows more and more wasteful?

Of course it is by no means only foreigners who are dismayed. A good many Americans, disturbed by our failure to win friends and influence people abroad, have come to think that we have, in effect,

sold our birthright for a very messy pottage, breeding an irresponsible race who litter our vacant lots and our national parks with equal spontaneity. We all feel self-consciously apologetic about this untidiness at times, especially just after we have read the latest best-selling indictment of our culture (usually referred to as "mass culture" nowadays) or just after we have returned from a trip abroad. In such moods we look about at the spasmodic cyclones of gum wrappers on subway platforms, at the sodden banks of garbage between which rivers of industrial waste flow to the sea, at the beer cans strewn along the shoulders of our highways, and we think wistfully of a scrubbed village square in Holland, the poplar-lined embankments of a river in Normandy, or a mathematically clean autobahn in Germany. It would be nice, we think, if America were not so unkempt.

Sometimes we feel the same way about our politics. Back in the 1920's, for example, when we got a glimpse of the political sewage flowing through Harding's Washington, some of us talked enviously of the disciplined efficiency of Mussolini's new regime in Italy. Not that we wanted Fascism, of course, even if the trains did run on time; but the idea of political discipline has its charms when you look at the disorderly machinery of democratic politics.

It is not only our political machinery that is messy; that of our industrial system is frequently

messy too. The teams of British technicians, workers, and managers who came here after the war, sponsored by the Anglo-American Productivity Council, were frequently struck by the untidiness of our factories and machines. As one report phrased it: "We found the standard of cleanliness of machines to be lower in America than in Britain. The attitude toward machinery cleaning in America seems to be that it is largely unproductive." But, having noted this, the report went on to say—in words reminiscent of some of Lincoln Steffens's remarks about our political machines—that there was "certainly no evidence that the dirtier machines were working any less efficiently" than the others.

That comment, it seems to me, evokes a paradox which underlies many aspects of our civilization. There are several ways in which the paradox can be stated, but they all add up to something like: "Waste not; have not" or "Nothing succeeds like a mess."

However you state it, it sounds as if it were flippant nonsense; but I suspect it is a clue to our history, nevertheless. And if it is, we had better look seriously at it; for these are times when an understanding of the dynamic of American experience matters a great deal—to our own confidence in ourselves and to others' confidence in us and in the things we profess to stand for.

Who Owns the Joint?

One way to get at the nature of the paradox of waste and abundance is to speculate a bit about the beer can by the highway, which at night picks up the beams from your car's headlights and glows like a panther's eye. Does it mean anything more than that we are a wasteful and untidy people?

Bearing in mind the oft-repeated charge that we are a people who waste a great deal of our wealth and talent upon packages, labels, and surfaces generally, and too little on what is inside; and further remembering that beer cans, like most of our packages for food and drink, are handsome, well made, and attractive; isn't the discarded can, glowing by the roadside, a witness of a countervailing contempt for packaging? Someone who had finished its contents threw it there without a thought, just to be rid of it.

But, it will be objected, the discarded can is also a sign of other kinds of contempt: contempt for natural beauty, and contempt for the rights of others to enjoy that beauty. Perhaps so; but we need not leap too inconsiderately to those conclusions. May it not be simply a sign that the person who tossed it there inhabits a world ungrooved by routine, a world in which he can be so mobile that he need not worry about that can blighting any landscape to which he is likely to return? As for the

other fellow's rights: if the man who tossed out the can does not mind other people's discarded beer cans—if, in fact, he rather likes the way they wink at him at night and show him the edge of the road— why should "the other fellow" object to his? Whose highway is it, anyway? And in a world where there is so much natural beauty, whole sierras full of it, whole Alleghenies full, what difference can a few beer cans by the highway make?

Frivolous as such questions may seem, I hope that they suggest that there is a rather tricky relationship between waste (symbolized by those beer cans) and abundance. Everyone enjoys the abundance which enables us to have so many beer cans to throw away, but many of us see no necessary connection between having them and tossing them indiscriminately out of car windows. What I am trying to suggest is that we may not be able to get rid of the mess without also getting rid of the abundance.

From one point of view, the relationship between abundance and waste is a simple one of cause and effect. If we did not have abundance we could not be wasteful. In other words, we are what Denis Brogan calls a people "who go away and leave things" because we have enough and to spare. If we did not, we would take those cans home with us, cut out their ends, slice the remaining tubes lengthwise, and roof our houses with them as the citizens of the depression's Hoovervilles did. If the

221

cause-and-effect relationship is all there is to it, we can make America a tidier and less wasteful place simply by getting rid of our abundance—by giving it away or reducing the efficiency of our productive system.

However, as the roadside beer can suggests, there are other things than a consciousness of abundance which may prompt the American to indulge in litter and waste. One is his mobility, and another is his sense that he is what Pearl Bailey elegantly calls "the character that owns the joint." Now, these are not necessarily the most admirable or endearing characteristics of the American, but they are linked to an element of our environment which is at least as important as abundance: namely, democracy, or at any rate that sort of democracy with which we Americans are familiar. And this raises the question whether waste (and consequent untidiness) may not be as much a result of democracy as of abundance.

There are many who think so; the wastefulness of democracy has frequently been asserted. In a recent book by a distinguished American historian it is flatly said, for example, that after two hundred years of democracy intelligent Americans are beginning to realize that its emphasis on mobility and its denial of status have been excessively wasteful.

A democracy, by definition, must promise people opportunity to improve their standard of living, to develop their individual potentialities, to rise in

222

the social scale, and so on; and that promise has the double effect of putting a premium on all kinds of mobility (social, economic, and geographical) and of requiring the rejection of any fixed system of hierarchical status, whereby individuals are assigned by birth or edict to graded ranks. By this insistence, the argument goes, democracy has bred frightful insecurity and destructive psychological tensions, thereby precipitating what Eric Fromm has called the "escape from freedom" and inducing that flight toward security which has bred the types described in Adorno's *The Authoritarian Personality*.

Dangers of the Closed Frontier

This was all very well, one gathers, as long as there were ample undeveloped resources which people could get by going after them. But now that the real frontiers are closed and we have only what Professor Walter Prescott Webb calls mirages of new frontiers to pursue; now that the unconverted potentialities of abundance have been all but exhausted, it is seriously urged that there is no longer any great need for mobility, and that we must now recapture some of the security that goes with status.

Impressed by such arguments, some Americans are beginning to feel that it is cruelly wasteful, if not socially dangerous, to educate everybody (as the principle of democracy requires us to do) without determining in advance whether there will

be jobs available in which they can use their education. Several years ago, at a dinner in honor of General Eisenhower when he was president of Columbia, the then chancellor of the New York State Board of Regents (the head of the state's system of public education) warned against educating more men and women than can earn a living in the field in which they have been educated, lest they "turn upon" the society which aroused expectations that could not be fulfilled. What worried the chancellor especially was that these people would be "better armed in their destructive wrath by the education we have given them." If anyone was reminded of the slaveholders' reluctance to allow the slaves to learn to read and write, no comment was made.

But it is not only democracy's commitment to education which alarms such people. They are troubled too by the way it "encourages people to determine their own goals" and to set their own courses toward them, instead, presumably, of leaving goal-setting and course-plotting to what Ortega y Gasset calls "select and specially qualified minorities." What is the sense of letting people set goals for themselves which the limitations of a disfrontiered civilization will make it impossible for them to reach? The social waste resulting from this sort of thing seems, to some of those who believe themselves "qualified" to judge, too great for our civilization to bear.

From this point of view status now appears to

be something which society must assure, in order to relieve the tensions of insecurity. Hence "togetherness." Hence the widespread approval of the emphasis which the personnel officers of large corporations place upon giving employees a sense of membership in a permanent organization. Hence also the increasing emphasis in labor-union contracts—and in college contracts with the faculty—upon seniority, tenure, and pensions. Hence, furthermore, the popular interest in status variously reflected in such widely read books as Riesman's *The Lonely Crowd* and W. H. Whyte's *The Organization Man*.

From this point of view the beer can by the highway glows with a sinister light indeed, since it is a symbol both of mobility and of a far from reverent attitude toward the decorum of a status-oriented society.

The Goose and the Golden Egg

I do not view the beer can in that light. Those who do so seem to me to misconstrue the relationships between democracy, waste, and abundance. They assume that democracy is a by-product of abundance; that free land and plentiful natural resources are prerequisite to democracy. As for waste, that seems to them to be an undesirable by-product of both the other two. Since they also believe that the available supply of free land and natural resources is on the verge of being exhausted,

225

they regard waste of any kind as something which must be prevented.

I would argue, on the contrary, that a commitment to democracy—and a certain indifference to waste and untidiness—are prerequisite to abundance. I would argue, further, that we and others must learn this quickly because our ability to help create a peaceful world depends upon our ability to maintain our own abundance while helping others to create it for themselves.

By a "commitment to democracy" I mean a commitment to the idea that there are no fixed or determinable limits to the capacities of any individual human being, and that all are entitled, by inalienable right, to equal opportunities to develop their potentialities. Democracy in this sense is an ideal, not a political system, and certainly not an actual state of affairs.

But in order that we may understand one another, let us agree that the term "a democracy" means any set of political, economic, and social institutions, anywhere in the world, which has been shaped primarily under the influence of the ideal of democracy, no matter how much one such set of institutions may differ from others because of local conditions. If, as I think, American institutions have been shaped by the democratic ideal to a greater degree than those of some other nations, that is only because they were established at a time when the democratic ideal was in the ascendancy

in the Western world; in a place where there were no already-established institutions which conflicted with or were hostile to democracy; and by people who, having been chiefly "the poor and down-trodden of Western Europe," had little reason to be attached to the non-democratic or anti-democratic institutions still dominant in many areas of European life.

There can be no dispute, I think, about the fact that the two nations which, during the past two centuries, have most successfully converted potential abundance into actual abundance have been the two nations whose political, social, and economic institutions were most fully shaped by democratic ideals: namely, Great Britain and the United States. The only question is whether their success in creating abundance accounts for their having been able to achieve democratic institutions, or whether the attitudes toward man, nature, and God which are embodied in the democratic ideal made it possible for their people to create the unprecedented abundance which they have enjoyed. In other words, which came first, the goose or the golden egg?

The question is important, to us and to all the world, because men everywhere seem to have an insatiable appetite for golden eggs, and one way or another they are determined to get some—by fighting for them if necessary. In so far as we believe that the golden eggs come first, our domestic and

foreign policy will consist in efforts to distribute the present stock of eggs equitably enough to keep the hunger for them in check. In so far as we are convinced that the democratic goose comes first, we will do what we can to encourage the growth of any goslings we can discern (whether in Iran, or Indonesia, or Spain, or Russia)—not insisting that they grow up to be geese of exactly the same color and shape and size as ours, and not worrying very much how untidy (or how unimpressed by our status among world powers) they may be.

I am assuming, of course, that the democratic ideal exists, in at least the gosling state, wherever human beings exist, whether or not there are any golden eggs in the neighborhood. It seems a reasonable assumption, since mankind created and cherished the legend of the goose that laid the golden eggs many centuries before the realization of any such dream of abundance was even remotely conceivable. (It is worth noting that, even in the fantasy-world of the legend, the possessor of the goose kills it—as if men couldn't quite allow themselves to attain abundance even in their dreams.)

Certainly the ideal of democracy long antedates the existence of any abundance-creating civilization. Historians are apparently agreed that economic insufficiency characterized all civilizations until quite recent times—say about two centuries ago at the earliest. In all civilized nations up to that time a majority of the people were "inescapably

destined to heavy toil and bare subsistence," since the economic surplus was insufficient to provide leisure and abundance for more than a very small minority.

In such circumstances the enviable minority had to keep the ideal of democracy in check if order was to be preserved. To them this would seem neither selfish nor heartless, but plain common sense. Feeling, like all human beings, that the maximum development of human potentialities was an unqualified good, and knowing that it required some leisure and abundance, they naturally wished to retain what advantages they themselves had. They might be (and probably were, at times) sorry for those who did not have it, and might even give some of their surplus away to those whose deprivation was called to their attention. But it must have been clear to them that it was from men and women of their privileged group—not from the lower orders—that one could expect those achievements in the arts, sciences, and professions which most fully revealed the wonderful resources of man's nature. And they must have felt quite justified in trying to avert or stamp out any activity among the vast majority of people which threatened the economic basis of their capacity to enjoy and to exalt humanity's finest potentialities.

To them a system of subordination transmitted by heredity would naturally seem less wasteful and more orderly than one which would—as democratic

systems do—conduct what Professor David Potter has called "a great social steeplechase for the purpose of selecting a handful of winners to occupy a few enviable positions." A system of fixed status had the undeniable merit of giving everybody a secure sense that he knew where he belonged and what was expected of him. (It is more than a coincidence, I suspect, that the first issue of *Who's Who*—a reference book which would be of no possible use in a society which knew who who was—appeared in England the year after the revolutionary turmoils of 1848.)

Besides, in a relatively static society with a limited economic surplus, no one had more than a statistically negligible chance for advancement, even if the social steeplechase had been permitted. And even if the hereditary ruling class sometimes had unruly and inconsequential sons, there probably did not seem to be any urgent necessity to recruit new blood from the depressingly underfed, undereducated, and overworked majority. Annoying expressions of hunger for a golden egg could be disposed of by promises of utopia in some distant future, or by such relatively inexpensive distractions as Rome's "bread and circuses" or, later, state lotteries; or at worst by the provision of enough governmental or private charity to silence the most insistent complaints.

The trouble was that, all the while that the very human need to develop one's maximum poten-

tialities was admonishing the privileged few to hold onto what they had, the very same need was constantly fermenting among those who had little. Every now and then some exceptional, or exceptionally lucky, individual rose out of the anonymous mass and got a share of the surplus. Once he had more than the bare necessities, the dynamics of his talent and energy impelled him to disrupt, to a greater or less extent, the relatively fixed status of those at the top.

They, on the other hand, when faced with the energies of a Shakespeare, a Martin Luther, a Napoleon, reacted too late or too sluggishly to preserve unaltered the institutions which such upstarts challenged; with the result that hierarchical institutions in every area of life were forever being modified by pressures from below. For it is axiomatic that security of status, accompanied by abundance, tends to be relaxing. Those who possess it easily succumb to the illusion of permanence. They find it soothing to believe that change, instead of meaning a continuous process of development (and concomitant waste), means only five nickels for a quarter—which is still twenty-five cents. And so, though the process of development and waste goes inexorably on—in human affairs as it does throughout nature—those at the top of the social hierarchy are relatively insulated from the changes which the process inevitably produces.

The upward pressures in Western European civ-

ilization had accumulated irresistible force by about 1500. The rapid advances in technology after that time—the swift development of power-driven machines—culminated in the so-called industrial revolution of the late eighteenth and early nineteenth centuries. And that revolution brought abundance within reach of the majority of people for the first time in the history of civilization.

The Brace-and-Bit and All That

It is precisely at this point that we run head on into the question whether the goose or the golden egg came first. Professor Webb's theory of the Great Frontier, as applied to Western civilization in general—like Turner's earlier thesis about the role of the frontier in American history—rests on the assumption that it was the discovery and pre-emption of vast areas of unused land which suddenly made abundance available on an unprecedented scale, thereby creating conditions favorable to the development of those institutions and qualities of character (including self-reliant individualism) which we associate with democracy. Similarly, Professor Potter has argued (in his influential book, *People of Plenty*) that free land was only one aspect of a total increase of natural resources which—combined with a flourishing technology—produced abundance enough to enable men to afford democracy. Both theories by implication suggest that a sudden in-

crease in wealth was, in effect, the golden egg tossed by fate into the lap of Western man, and that only after men had the golden egg were they able or willing to fatten the democratic goose.

The frontier theory has stimulated some brilliant historical writing, notably Professor Webb's splendid books, and its grand sweep has a tragic persuasiveness. But a skeptical reader is bound to ask why, for example, if the western prairies and plains made the Americans "democratic, prosperous, and numerous," as Turner maintained, they did not have a similar effect upon the Indians, or (as George Wilson Pierson more pertinently asked) upon the Spaniards whose frontier they were before they were ours.

Similarly, if internal social forces in Europe in Luther's time were dynamic enough to cause a religious revolution, one wonders why the stimulus from an external frontier was necessary to incite a technical revolution. Actually—as Lynn White, Jr., and other historians of medieval technology have recently shown—there is a good deal of evidence that the technical revolution was well under way before the Great Frontier of the New World was discovered. The spinning wheel—a key invention of modern technology—dates from about A.D. 1300, and by 1420 an anonymous carpenter or shipwright, probably in Flanders, had invented the brace-and-bit, thereby inventing the compound crank (familiar to you in the form of the crankshaft in your auto-

mobile engine) and precipitating what is probably the greatest single revolution in the design of machines. By 1430—sixty years before Columbus—Western man had built machines involving double compound cranks with two connecting rods and was on the way to a Model-T and a Cadillac.

But there are other reasons for doubting that free land is the cause of either democracy or abundance. It was Spain, not England, which first had direct access to the New World's wealth in its most easily convertible form—gold and silver; but it was England which became the breeding ground of democratic institutions. In our own country, New England in the nineteenth century was relatively poor in natural resources while the South was relatively rich—but it was New England which developed the technology and productivity to make abundance available while the more "aristocratic" South contributed almost nothing to the development of technology and became one of the poorest regions in the nation.

These and many similar instances suggest, I think, that the golden egg is not immaculately conceived or doled out in a cosmic lottery, but is engendered like other eggs and, like them, must be fertilized. There may be no conclusive proof that democracy was in fact the goose that laid the golden egg of abundance, but the evidence with which I am familiar certainly makes it seem probable.

Who Gets Ahead?

It would be foolish, of course, to underestimate
the role of technology in creating abundance. No
one need be so naïve as to believe that all you need
in order to be rich is to be a good democrat. So, also,
it is true that there is a relationship between technology and natural resources. Professor Webb is
clearly right in saying that industrial machinery
cannot exist "apart from a body of material to be
fabricated." But it does not necessarily follow that
"it was the great abundance of raw material which
put a high premium on improving the tools" of
technology, and that it was this high premium, in
turn, which fostered the ingenuity, inventiveness,
and other traits necessary to produce a system of
abundance. If that were so, the ante-bellum South
would have outstripped Vermont and Connecticut
in developing machines, and the Georgia cracker,
not the Yankee, would have been inventive and
mechanically adaptable.

It can be much more plausibly argued that people who are inventive, ingenious, and in other respects mobile are more likely than those who relish
or depend upon security of status to recognize potential abundance when they see it. They also are
more likely to assume that even though no one ever
tried to convert a given resource into actual wealth
before, it can probably be done. Furthermore, there

is a great deal of evidence that a relative paucity of resources, rather than abundance, encourages the improvement of machines and tools. For instance, it was only after wood began to become scarce that we bothered to perfect mechanical saws which didn't produce almost as many pounds of sawdust as of lumber. All the evidence, I think, points to the conclusion that inventiveness, adaptability, and other qualities which tend to foster industrial productivity (and hence abundance) are directly traceable to drives inherent in the democratic ideal, drives which are nourished by political, economic, and social institutions—and I specifically mean to include religious institutions—which are shaped by that ideal.

In this connection it is worth noting that the reports of those Productivity Teams sent over from Britain after the war give no evidence that high productivity shows any correlation with abundance of natural resources or with the security of a system of fixed status. On the contrary, the reports are full of evidence, explicit and implied, that mobility—and the institutions which foster it—are the chief factors in making America's industrial system more productive than that even of Britain, which in turn is far more productive than that of France, let us say, or of Latin America. This evidence is adduced by observers who had no motive for wanting or expecting American institutions to emerge in such a favorable light. Over and over, in these reports, there are remarks to the

effect that Americans "accept new machines, new methods, and the use of new materials more readily than their British counterparts"; or that the Americans are more willing than the British "to put opportunity before security."

All this may sound terribly out-of-date and other-worldly at a time when the Russians have made such spectacular advances in the conquest of outer space. If technology is fostered by democratic institutions, how did the Russians get ahead of us? The answer, of course, is that an autocratically directed technology can do almost anything for which it is willing to sacrifice enough. Hitler's Germany proved as much, as did the Kaiser's before it. But the Kaiser's tanks and Hitler's V-1 and V-2 rockets and Khrushchev's sputniks were not abundance, and the productivity of an autocratically directed technology has never yet equaled that of the democracies. Some of us are now so frightened that we think maybe this time it will.

"Belonging" to What?

I do not mean to underestimate the importance of security. I know the psychological damage which may result from excessive insecurity, or from living in an environment which seems at times to frustrate us at every turn. The point I am concerned to make is simply that some of the current assumptions about the relationships between democracy and abun-

dance, mobility and waste, lead to what seem to me to be fundamental misconceptions about what we must do. They lead to fruitless attempts to eliminate insecurity by providing makeshift substitutes for obsolete systems of status, instead of taking advantage of opportunities—inherent in democratic mobility—to minimize the sense of insecurity and to maximize the transmuting possibilities of change.

The aversion to mobility and change, in our time as in the past, springs from fear. They seem to threaten the abundance which now enables us to divert our energies from mere subsistence into channels of creative endeavor and spiritual development. Men individually, and men corporately as nations, are still driven by this inner necessity to realize their human potentialities. They will go to almost any lengths to ward off a threat to those advantages they have already won.

Since an economic surplus is one of the most recently achieved of these advantages, and since even now the vast numbers who lack it remind us of the way in which poverty can warp and dwarf the human spirit, we inevitably set a high value on abundance. The materialism of modern civilization, in this light, seems understandable enough. And if, besides seeming so desirable, abundance seems to us to be something of which there is a fixed and limited supply, it is scarcely surprising that mobility and waste will seem dangerous, while the ideals of

status and order (and the hierarchical institutions which reinforce those ideals) will have a renewed appeal.

We must learn that the craving for status is, at bottom, only the human need for a sense of belonging. Historically, this sense of belonging has been associated with a hierarchy of fixed classes, and with the handicrafts and agricultural techniques appropriate to a status-oriented society. We tend, therefore, to overlook the evidence (of which there is a great deal) that one can belong, and have the sense of belonging, to a process as well as to a class. The awareness of process is new, and the institutions of our mobile society—including its religious and educational institutions—are still bedeviled by leftover preconceptions from an earlier order. Consequently, many of us are convinced that the only kind of belonging that matters is belonging to a cozily defined class, be it the "Workers," or the "Upper Bohemians," or the "Eggheads," or some other sociological Sigma Chi whose sweetheart we can be. It is understandable enough, to be sure, but it may well be suicidal.

Fifty Poor Melons

As for the contemporary dread of wastefulness, so eloquently witnessed by the current interest in conservation, it too is frequently linked with the notion of rigidly limited resources. Writing in

the *American Scientist* not long ago, Paul B. Sears asked whether human beings can continue to increase not only their numbers but also "their individual needs, their range and speed" without having to come to terms with "the limitations of a finite environment" as other organisms do. Of course his answer, based upon his ecological research and broad experience in the field of conservation, was that they cannot, even in America—because, vast as our resources and space may be, they "still are certainly finite."

Leaving aside the question whether the conquest of space can remove the finite limitations upon resources—and accepting wholeheartedly the ideal of respect for all forms of organic and inorganic nature—I would only point out the danger that, in times of apprehension, a legitimate interest in averting wanton destruction of resources may degenerate into an equally wasteful passion for hoarding them. Conservation may become mere parsimony, and in the name of the love of nature we may become nature's slaves, instead of her partners. We need occasionally to be reminded of the spirit in which the first great American conservationist, George P. Marsh, worked and wrote. If man is destined to inhabit the world much longer, and to continue to advance, he said almost a century ago, he will have to learn not only to put "a wiser estimate on the works of creation" but also to profit materially "from stimulating [nature's] productive ener-

gies in provinces of her empire hitherto regarded as forever inaccessible, utterly barren."

We must learn, what nature can surely teach us, that abundance is in a sense a product of waste. As Emerson said many years ago, "nature makes fifty poor melons for one that is good . . . and she scatters nations of naked Indians, and nations of clothed Christians, with two or three good heads among them. Nature works very hard, and only hits the white once in a million throws."

With his reiterated insistence upon "the infinitude of the private man," Emerson is not in high favor in these days of "togetherness" and "the organization man." Yet it might be good for us to look for a moment through his eyes at the abundant and wasteful civilization in which we live.

Looking about him at the American scene near the end of his life, he observed that—in spite of the European economists' doleful allegiance to the idea that the condition of the great body of the people is fated to be, since it always has been, generally poor and miserable—that same "great body" here in America had arrived at "a sloven plenty . . . an unbuttoned comfort, not clean, not thoughtful, far from polished." It was, Emerson knew, an unprecedented condition, and the rules to meet it were not set down "in any history." What we needed, he concluded, were men and women "of original perception and original action, who can open their eyes wider than to a nationality,—namely to considera-

tions of benefit to the human race . . . ; men of elastic, men of moral mind, who can live in the moment and take a step forward."

We need such people more than ever now. And I think that it is from men and women who share Emerson's open-ended conception of man's potentialities—which is the root and seed of democracy—that we will get that open-ended conception of abundance, that refusal to accept limits to potential wealth or virtue or kindness or talent, which will enable us to keep all doors open to our own self-fulfillment while helping others to open doors for themselves.

ACKNOWLEDGMENTS

As THE DEDICATION SUGGESTS, this book owes a great deal to Joan Vatsek Kouwenhoven, my wife. If the essays as they are printed here have a clarity they did not possess in their earlier forms, and if they are more consistent with one another in their present juxtaposition than they were, it is primarily because she resolutely pestered me to say, if possible, exactly what I meant instead of merely taking a stab at it and because she has a delightfully meddlesome way of recognizing inconsistencies when she encounters them.

Most of the essays have been published before, often under different titles and usually in considerably different form. The notes at the bottom of each essay's title page indicate its provenance, but do not suggest the degree to which I am generally indebted to the editors of the magazines and the sponsors of the pamphlets in which they were published and to the institutions and individuals who, by asking me to give lectures or addresses, have forced me to grapple with ideas and impressions which would otherwise have floated around helter-

skelter. Nor do they indicate my indebtedness, through reading and conversation, to the stimulation of many other minds—both those whose perceptions seemed to me, when I encountered them, to be anticipations of what I was about to say, and those whose views acted as abrasives upon which I could sharpen my own.

Those to whom I am most vividly aware of my indebtedness in these essays include the students who have worked with me at Barnard College and a number of my colleagues on the faculty at Barnard and Columbia, especially my fellow members of the University Seminar on American Civilization. I owe a curiously non-specifiable debt to the Carnegie Corporation, and its president, John W. Gardner, for having allowed me to vegetate for a year as the recipient of the first of their "Reflective Year" Fellowships, during which time some of the ideas in these essays germinated. My intellectual debt to several writers is suggested but inadequately acknowledged by my references in the essays to their work.

In addition I gratefully acknowledge the stimulus and help I have at different times, over the past ten years, received from individuals who have been interested in my work, including: my former wife, Eleanor Hayden Kouwenhoven; Alexander Girard; Thomas Hornsby Ferril; James Marston Fitch; Eric Larrabee; Frederick G. Frost, Jr., and his son Corwin Frost; Lynn White, Jr.; Dean and

Acknowledgments

Virginia Rusk; John R. Frazier; Walter Prescott Webb; Russell Lynes; Leo Leonni; Robert E. Alexander; James Real; and my editor at Doubleday, Samuel S. Vaughan.

INDEX

Date Due